Role of Microbes in Human Health and Diseases

Edited by Nar Singh Chauhan

Published in London, United Kingdom

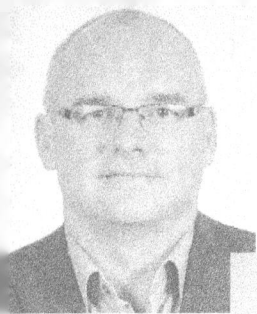
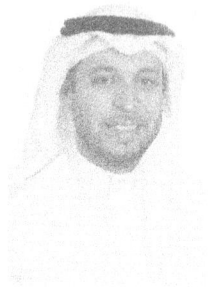
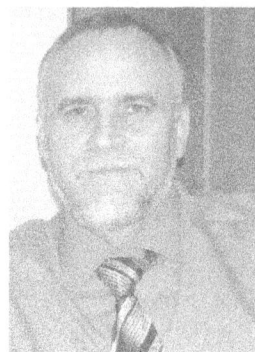
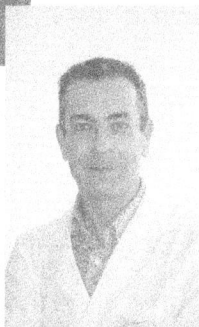
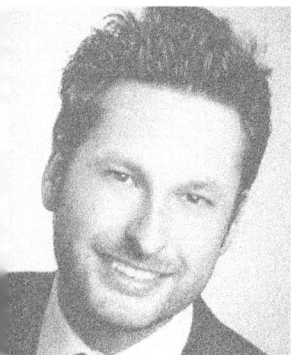
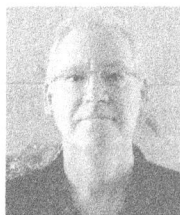
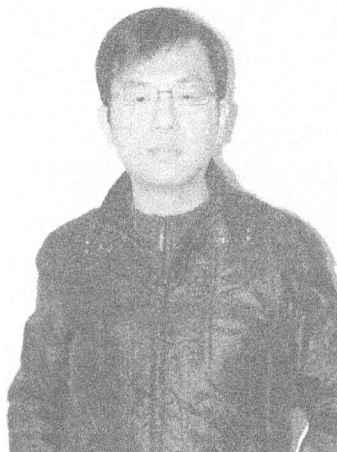

IntechOpen

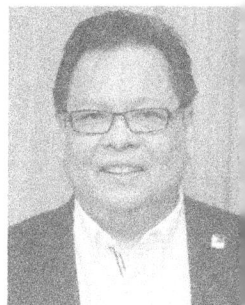
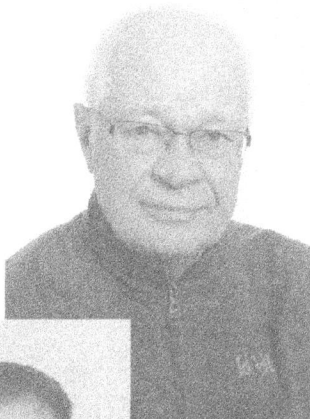
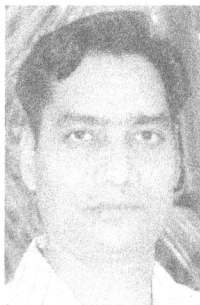
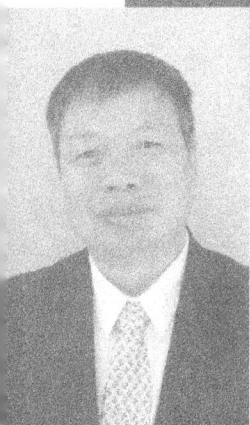
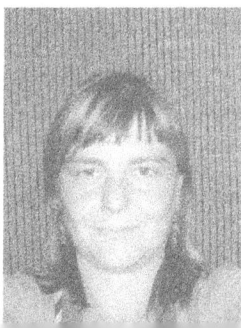
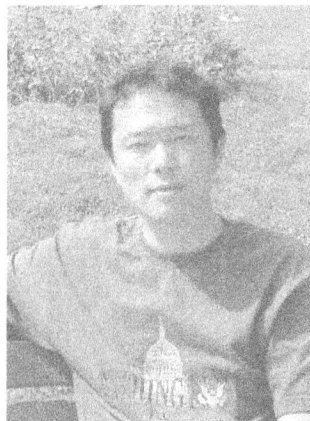

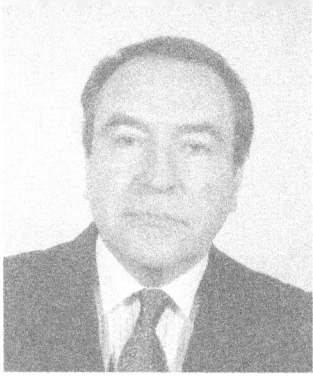

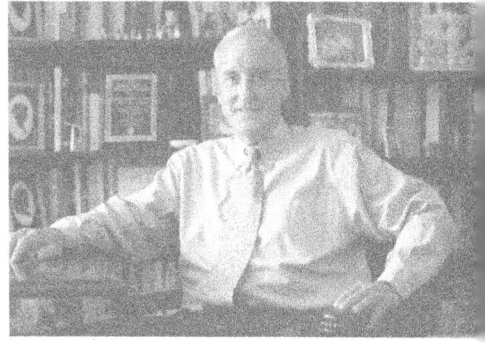

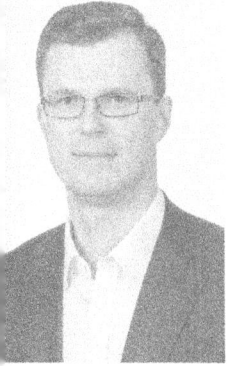

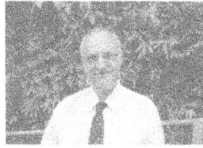

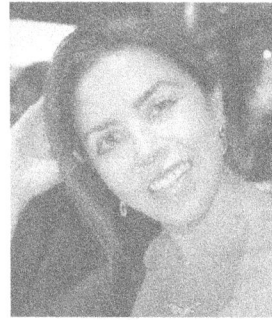

Supporting open minds since 2005

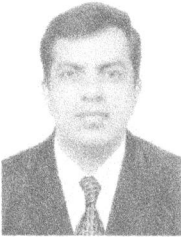

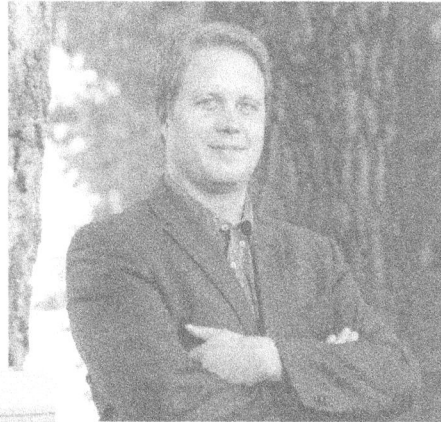

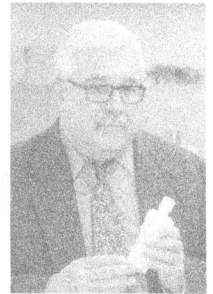

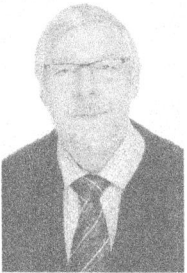

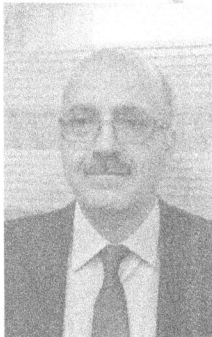

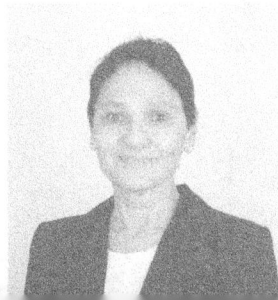

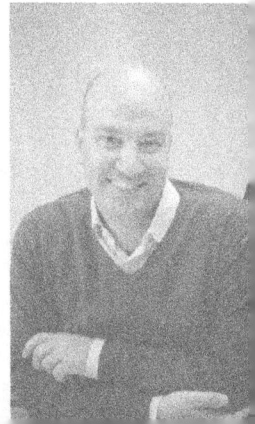

Role of Microbes in Human Health and Diseases
http://dx.doi.org/10.5772/intechopen.76595
Edited by Nar Singh Chauhan

Contributors
Onix Cantres-Fonseca, William Rodriguez-Cintrón, Francisco Del Olmo, Stella Baez-Corujo,
Shabarinath Srikumar, Richard Oruko, John Odiyo, Joshua Edokpayi, Nar Singh Chauhan

Notice
Statements and opinions expressed in the chapters are these of the individual contributors and not
necessarily those of the editors or publisher. No responsibility is accepted for the accuracy of
information contained in the published chapters. The publisher assumes no responsibility for any
damage or injury to persons or property arising out of the use of any materials, instructions, methods
or ideas contained in the book.

First published in London, United Kingdom, 2019 by IntechOpen
IntechOpen is the global imprint of INTECHOPEN LIMITED, registered in England and Wales,
registration number: 11086078, The Shard, 25th floor, 32 London Bridge Street
London, SE19SG – United Kingdom
Printed in Croatia

British Library Cataloguing-in-Publication Data
A catalogue record for this book is available from the British Library

Additional hard and PDF copies can be obtained from orders@intechopen.com

Role of Microbes in Human Health and Diseases
Edited by Nar Singh Chauhan
p. cm.
Print ISBN 978-1-83880-233-2
Online ISBN 978-1-83880-234-9
eBook (PDF) ISBN 978-1-83880-718-4

We are IntechOpen,
the world's leading publisher of
Open Access books
Built by scientists, for scientists

4,200+
Open access books available

116,000+
International authors and editors

125M+
Downloads

Our authors are among the

151
Countries delivered to

Top 1%
most cited scientists

12.2%
Contributors from top 500 universities

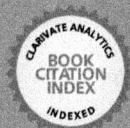

CLARIVATE ANALYTICS
BOOK
CITATION
INDEX
INDEXED

WEB OF SCIENCE™

Selection of our books indexed in the Book Citation Index
in Web of Science™ Core Collection (BKCI)

Interested in publishing with us?
Contact book.department@intechopen.com

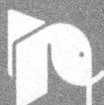

Meet the editor

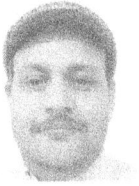

Dr. Nar Singh Chauhan is currently a teaching faculty in the Department of Biochemistry, Maharishi Dayanand University, Rohtak, India. His doctor of philosophy degree, with thesis research on "Arsenic detoxification mechanisms in unculturable bacteria using function metagenomics" at the CSIR-Institute of Genomics and Integrative Biology, was granted by Savitribai Phule Pune University, Pune, India. His current research focus is on the metagenomic characterization of diverse microbiome for their native community structure, physiological functions, survival strategies under abiotic stress, colonization factors, and host-microbial interactions. In this direction, he has established an association of the human microbiome with the onset of celiac disease and chronic obstructive pulmonary disease. Dr. Chauhan is the author of a number of peer-reviewed research publications in reputed international journals (*Genome Biology & Evolution*, *Scientific Reports*, *Frontiers in Microbiology*, etc.) and has also been awarded many research patents.

Contents

Preface

The human body is colonized by a vast number of microorganisms that live on and in humans, which are collectively called the "human microbiome." The scientific expedition to define the human microbiome started with the efforts of Antonie van Leewenhoek to compare oral and fecal microbiota in 1680. Since then, several attempts have been made to identify the role of microbes in human health and in the onset of infectious diseases. A number of discoveries have been made to identify, classify, and characterize microbes responsible for host health and the onset of diseases, factors affecting their pathogenicity, microbial physiology during the onset of diseases, as well as the role of antibiotic resistance in survivability. Simultaneously, it was found that the number of microbes defining the human microbiome was almost tenfold higher than human cells, which collectively codes for approximately 3.3 million genes compared to ~22,000 host-encoded genes. These outcomes redefine the human body as a "supraorganism" harboring a vast collection of microbial and human cells working in close coordination for a healthy host physiology. This book is aimed at providing an overview of the role of microbes in human health and diseases, the functional role of microbes in the maintenance of human health, and various scientific discoveries made to answer questions such as "what are human commensals and pathogens?", "how can a disequilibrium in microbiome structure lead to the onset of diseases?", and "how can the human microbiome function and negotiate with pathogenic microbes to prevent diseases?" I hope this book will enrich the knowledge domain of readers and answer their questions on the human microbiome and its function in host health and diseases.

Nar Singh Chauhan
Department of Biochemistry,
Maharshi Dayanand University,
Rohtak, Haryana, India

Section 1

Introduction

Chapter 1

Introductory Chapter: Human and Microbes in Health and Diseases

Nar Singh Chauhan

1. Introduction

Microbes are ubiquitous in nature and humans are no exception. Microbes have coevolved with humans and reside in and on human body to develop a host associated structure, called "Human Microbiome" or "Human Microbiota." These microbial counterparts account toward 10% of human body weight and outnumber human cells by approximately by tenfold and considered as commensals. Human microbiome is defined as the total genomes of microbes (constitute bacteria, bacteriophage, fungi, protozoa and viruses) that live inside or on the human body [1]. There are trillions of microbes living in/on human body plays a fundamental role in normal functioning of metabolic, physiological and immune system. Microbiota is a complex ecosystem consisting of bacteria, protozoa, viruses and fungi; all varies in number even in body parts of same individual. Human body has 10 times more bacteria than the number of human cells in our body [2]. Most of these bacteria are present in gastrointestinal tract [3] which account for approximate 70% of the total microbial load in or on human body (particular in large intestine) [4]. Humans are born sterile and start acquiring human companion to shape resilient microbiome structure. Establishment of microbiome starts with birth and matures with age. Microbial introduction and the establishment of microbiome is a random process influenced by many factor like mode of delivery, diet, sex, age, genetics, geographical location have a strong impact in shaping human microbiome structure [5–10]. These microbes are in symbiotic relationship, beside gut they are also found in mouth, respiratory tract, vagina and skin.

2. Human and microbes

The study of human microbiome diversity started with Antonie Van Leeuwenhoek, when he had a comparison of his oral and fecal microbiota in 1680s. He found that different microbes are present in different habitats and also different microbes are present in healthy and diseased person [11, 12]. There is a growing evidence that any change in microbiota composition leads to several metabolic diseases including obesity, diabetes and cardiovascular. Different parts of intestinal tract have different composition of microbes and it varies according to age, weight, site and diet. Composition of microbiota in gut alters by nutrition, drugs, diet and genetic background and lifestyle. Microbiota regulates metabolic and physiological mechanisms by producing metabolites. It has been found out that different species of microbiota in gut works under same metabolic pathway [9]. Qualitative and quantitative alteration in gut microbiota leads to dysbiosis by consuming antibiotics, physical and psychological stress [13]. Recent studies shows evidence regarding change in composition by urban and rural environment, affects skin (allergic symptoms) of particular organisms. Age alter the environmental effects on individual such as alter microbiota variations in skin between children and teenager cause skin allergies [14]. Microbiome structure varies in respect of host anatomical and physiological sites. Normally, flora found in/on the body surface in stable condition to compete with pathogenic microbes in environment or those microbes entered in specific body parts [15]. As in addition to these permanent residents, a number of microbes known as causative agent for various infectious diseases. Likewise commensals, these infectious agents have evolved an efficient machinery to evade host protective gears for their successful proliferation in various anatomical locations. Normal bacteria defend host against the invasion of pathogenic microorganisms by inducing barrier against them [16]. It was observed that host commensals plays a critical role in balancing the abundance of pathogenic and nonpathogenic microbial strains and protects the host form the onset of any infectious diseases. However a number of factors like change in diet, variable host immune response, fluctuating environmental conditions like pH, oxygen saturation, ionic strength, etc., could induce microbial dysbiosis and induce microbial community dynamics. These microbial community dynamics could induce favorable conditions for growth of earlier dormant pathogenic microbes and result in onset of infectious diseases [16].

3. Conclusion

Microbes have been identified to play a vital role in human health and diseases. Physiological characterization of these microbes and defining their functional molecular machinery could enable us to develop potential therapeutic and diagnostic targets. Additionally, holistic overview of human microbiome structure, human microbe interactions and role of microbes in human health and diseases are the key areas of current research focus. In-depth information about host microbial interaction in human health and diseases could enable to identify causative factors for development of host physiological/metabolic disorders. Current book comprises of various chapters defining a relation among human and microbes in health and diseases.

Author details

Nar Singh Chauhan
Department of Biochemistry, Maharshi Dayanand University, Rohtak, Haryana, India

*Address all correspondence to: nschauhanmdu@gmail.com

IntechOpen

References

[1] Xu J. Invited review: Microbial ecology in the age of genomics and metagenomics: Concepts, tools, and recent advances. Molecular Ecology. 2006;**15**(7):1713-1731

[2] Sender R, Fuchs S, Milo R. Revised estimates for the number of human and bacteria cells in the body. PLoS Biology. 2016;**14**(8):e1002533

[3] Zoetendal EG, von Wright A, Vilpponen-Salmela T, Ben-Amor K, Akkermans AD, de Vos WM. Mucosa-associated bacteria in the human gastrointestinal tract are uniformly distributed along the colon and differ from the community recovered from feces. Applied and Environmental Microbiology. 2002;**68**(7):3401-3407

[4] Turnbaugh PJ, Hamady M, Yatsunenko T, Cantarel BL, Duncan A, Ley RE, et al. A core gut microbiome in obese and lean twins. Nature. 2009;**457**(7228):480

[5] David LA, Maurice CF, Carmody RN, Gootenberg DB, Button JE, Wolfe BE, et al. Diet rapidly and reproducibly alters the human gut microbiome. Nature. 2014;**505**(7484):559-563. DOI: 10.1038/nature12820

[6] Chu DM, Ma J, Prince AL, Antony KM, Seferovic MD, Aagaard KM. Maturation of the infant microbiome community structure and function across multiple body sites and in relation to mode of delivery. Nature Medicine. 2017;**23**:314-326. DOI: 10.1038/nm.4272

[7] Dominianni C, Sinha R, Goedert JJ, Pei Z, Yang L, Hayes RB, et al. Sex, body mass index, and dietary fiber intake influence the human gut microbiome. PLoS One. 2015;**10**(4):e0124599. DOI: 10.1371/journal.pone.0124599. eCollection 2015

[8] Jakobsson HE, Abrahamsson TR, Jenmalm MC, Harris K, Quince C, Jernberg C, et al. Decreased gut microbiota diversity, delayed bacteroidetes colonisation and reduced Th1 responses in infants delivered by caesarean section. Gut. 2013;**63**(4):559-566. DOI: 10.1136/gutjnl-2012-303249

[9] Joice R, Yasuda K, Shafquat A, Morgan XC, Huttenhower C. Determining microbial products and identifying molecular targets in the human microbiome. Cell Metabolism. 2014;**20**(5):731-741. DOI: 10.1016/j.cmet.2014.10.003

[10] Milan AM, Cameron-Smith D. Digestion and postprandial metabolism in the elderly. Advances in Food and Nutrition Research. 2015;**76**:79-124

[11] Dobell C. The discovery of the intestinal protozoa of man. Proceedings of the Royal Society of Medicine. 1920;**13**(Sect_Hist_Med):1-15

[12] Van Leeuwenhoek A. An abstract of a letter from Antonie van Leeuwenhoek. About animals in the scrurf of the teeth. Philosophical Transactions of the Royal Society of London. 1683;**14**:568-574

[13] Ley RE, Peterson DA, Gordon JI. Ecological and evolutionary forces shaping microbial diversity in the human intestine. Cell. 2006;**124**:837-848

[14] Ley RE, Bäckhed F, Turnbaugh P, Lozupone CA, Knight RD, Gordon JI. Obesity alters gut microbial ecology. Proceedings of the National Academy of Sciences. 2005;**102**(31):11070-11075

[15] Faust K, Sathirapongsasuti JF, Izard J, Segata N, Gevers D, Raes J, et al. Microbial co-occurrence relationships in the human microbiome. PLoS Computational Biology. 2012;**8**(7):

e1002606. DOI: 10.1371/journal.
pcbi.1002606

[16] Littman DR, Pamer EG. Role of the
commensal microbiota in normal and
pathogenic host immune responses. Cell
Host & Microbe. 2011;**10**(4):311-323.
DOI: 10.1016/j.chom.2011.10.004

Section 2

Gut Microbes

Chapter 2

The Therapeutic Potential of the "Yin-Yang" Garden in Our Gut

Shabarinath Srikumar and Séamus Fanning

Abstract

The gut microbiota is made up of trillion microorganisms comprising bacteria, archaea, and eukaryota living in an intimate relationship with the host. This is a highly diverse microbial community and is essentially an open ecosystem despite being deeply embedded in the human body. The gut microbiome is continually exposed to allochthonous bacteria that primarily originates from food intake. Comprising more than 1000 bacterial species, the gut microbiota endows so many different functions—so many that can be considered as an endocrine organ of its own. In this book chapter, we summarize the importance of gut microbiota in the development and maintenance of a healthy human body. We first describe how the gut microbiota is formed during the birth of a human baby and how a healthy microflora is established overtime. We also discuss how important it is to maintain the microbiota in its homeostatic condition. A discussion is also given on how alterations in the microbiota are characteristic of many diseased conditions. Recent investigations report that reestablishing a healthy microbiota in a diseased individual using fecal microbial transplant can be used as a therapeutic approach in curing many diseases. We conclude this chapter with a detailed discussion on fecal microbial transplants.

Keywords: microbiome, microbiota, gut, antibiotic, IBD, FMT

1. Introduction

We, animals, live in a microbe-dominated planet. We are all covered, filled, and fueled by bacteria. All body surfaces like the skin, gastrointestinal tract, urogenital, and respiratory tract are in constant contact with the environment and are, therefore, colonized by bacteria. The realities of life associated with a microbe-dominated planet have led to the coevolution of animals with bacteria. This coevolution has led to close inhabitation of bacteria on different surfaces of the human body, especially the gut. Here, many bacteria and their phages, viruses, fungi, archaea, protists, and nematodes intermingle to form a microbial consortia collectively called "microbiome" or "microbiota". The presence and abundance of each taxonomic group may vary within population based on their access to adequate health care and local sanitation condition or within individuals based on their metabolic, medical, diet, and various other factors.

Despite being embedded deeply in the human body, the gut is essentially an open ecosystem—with constant exposure to environmental factors. The closure of the NIH-funded human microbiome project has given advanced understanding about the composition and functional characteristics of the gut microbiota composition. The composition of the human microbiome varies significantly depending on the habitat [1]. For example, the gut microbiota is mainly populated by bacteria [2], while the skin harbors mainly fungi [3]. It was always considered that human microbiome outnumbered human nucleated cells by at least a factor of 10. However, reports suggest that the ratio is closer to 1 [4]. Recently metagenomic analysis concluded that the gene set of the human microbiome is 150 times larger than the human gene complement raising the possibility that the large bacterial genetic repertoire aids the human component in performing the essential functions that are not encoded by the human genome. Since more than 99% of these genes are bacterial in origin, the number of bacterial species were calculated to be around 1000–1150 bacterial species. The figures collectively emphasize the biological importance of the microbiome, and the genetic complement can be rightly considered as the second genome [2]. However, the taxonomic diversity of the gut microbiome notwithstanding, this chapter will deal only with the bacterial populations and all further references to gut microbiota means gut bacterial microbiota.

A typical human gut microbiota contains about 10^{14} bacteria and is made up of more than 1000 bacterial species [5, 6]. The human gut microbiota is composed of six bacterial phyla—*Firmicutes, Proteobacteria, Bacteroides, Fusobacteria, Actinobacteria*, and *Verrucomicrobia*. Of this, *Bacteroides* and *Firmicutes* occupy 70–90% of the total bacteria present in a healthy gut, while others are present in lower abundances [7]. Under healthy circumstances *Proteobacteria* and *Verrucomicrobia* members are also present but in lesser abundance [8]. The huge complexity and the variability of the microbiome make the determination of precise metabolic functions and the host-microbe cross talk very difficult. However, recent advances in deep sequencing and computational biology have contributed to large advances into understanding the unique biology of the gut microbiota and the subject is still in its infancy.

The functions bestowed by the bacterial gut flora are so enormous that it can be considered as an endocrine organ on its own [9]. It is well understood that the gut microbiota and their metabolites play important roles in host homeostasis, such as providing important nutrients like secondary bile salts and B/K group vitamins [10, 11], help in fermenting the otherwise indigestible complex plant carbohydrates such as dietary fibers into short-chain fatty acids (SCFA) [12], contributing to an effective intestinal epithelial barrier and activation of both innate/adaptive immune responses of the host [13]. In addition, the healthy gut microbiome drives intestinal development by promoting vascularization, villus thickening, mucosal surface widening, mucus production, cellular proliferation, and maintaining epithelial junctions [14–16]. The influence of the gut microbiota, either directly or indirectly, affects the physiology of most host organs even the brain [14, 17–20].

The taxonomic composition of the microbiota is very subtle—subject to change with variations in the diet [21], feeding time changes [22], sleep wake cycles, and even jet lag [23]. The unique taxonomic signature of the gut microbiota has to be strictly maintained for a healthy gut. Any disruption of the taxonomic composition of the gut could lead to conditions such as inflammatory bowel syndrome (IBS), asthma, obesity, metabolic syndrome, and cancer [24]. In some cases, resuscitation of the gut microbiota using probiotic bacteria like *Bifidobacteria* and *Lactobacillus* leads to the mitigation of gut inflammation consequently regaining health.

In this chapter, we will sequentially detail how the microbiota establishes itself in a human body, how minor or major variations in the gut microbiome introduces diseased conditions, and how the recent therapeutic approaches aimed at resuscitating the healthy microbiota can cure many dysbiotic microbiota-associated conditions.

2. Our internal garden—on how gut microbiota is planted and nurtured

How do we become colonized with gut microbiota? Where do we get our initial inoculum from and how does this initial inoculum proceed in to a well-flourished, well-established microbiota? The first step to understanding this is to identify the initial inoculum and how this inoculum develops into a the full-fledged adult ecosystem following a series of ecological succession steps.

2.1 The initial colonization

The most prevalent concept, and a very incorrect one, is that babies are borne sterile and after birth, the body becomes immediately colonized with microbes from the surrounding environment. Placental mammals such as humans are borne through a birth canal, which is colonized by microbes. A baby acquires its first inoculum from the birth canal. A healthy vaginal microbiota is composed of few bacterial species [25, 26] and is predominated by *Lactobacilli* [27]. Consequently, naturally borne babies acquire vaginal microbes like *Lactobacillus, Prevotella*, and *Sneathia* spp. [28]. The bacteria are present in the mouth, skin, and even in the meconium. Therefore, all neonates are colonized by essentially the same vaginally derived bacteria obtained vertically from the mother. Once this microbiota is established, the microbiota becomes highly differentiated depending on their ability to colonize different body sites. For example, in the gut, facultative anaerobes establish and reduce the environment [29]. This highly reduced environment facilitates the colonization of obligate anaerobes [30–33]. In addition, breastfeeding will also enrich vaginally acquired lactic-acid-producing bacteria in the baby's intestine [34]. From then on, it is the physiology of the host habitat that selects the community that becomes well adapted to colonize that particular habitat. For example, the physiochemical, immunological, and the diet play an important role in determining the microbial community that will colonize the small and large intestines. The host genotype also appeared to influence the composition of the gut microbiota [35].

Cesarean section babies, in contrast to vaginally borne babies, are dominated by skin-associated bacteria like *Staphylococcus, Corynebacterium*, and *Propionibacterium* spp. [28]. The *Staphylococcal*-rich microbiota could be obtained from the skin of the humans the baby is in contact with. The lack of a natural first inoculum in C-section babies affects the bacterial community in the GI tract [36, 37]. This variation from the naturally borne baby's microbiome will increase the susceptibility of the C-section babies to certain pathogens. For example, about 70% of the MRSA-caused skin infection happens to C-section babies. In addition, there is an additional risk to atopic diseases [38], allergies, and asthma [28, 39].

2.2 Development of the microbiota

The establishment, composition, and the density of the microbiome in the gastrointestinal (GI) tract depends on the biochemical factors like pH, oxygen gradient, antimicrobial peptides (AMPs), bile salts, etc. There is a pH gradient across the GI tract—lowest in the stomach and gradually increase to the terminal ileum, and a drop in caecum and increases toward the distal colon. Oxygen also exhibits a gradient across the length of the tract. The levels are highest in the upper GI tract, which decrease to anaerobic conditions in the distal colon. Radially across the tract too, there exists a oxygen gradient. Anoxic conditions exist in the lumen, while there is an increase in the oxygen tension near the mucosa, and this oxygen is rapidly consumed by the facultative anaerobes [40]. Each area in the gut produces its own AMPs. Saliva contains lysozyme, which is antibacterial. Small intestine produces α-defensins, C-type lectins, lysozyme, and phospholipase A2. The large intestine produces β-defensins, C-type lectins, cathelicidins, galectins, and lipocalin. Mucus also plays an important role in the distribution of the gut microbiota. The mucus in the stomach and colon can be discriminated into two layers—outer loose layer, which is densely populated by bacteria, and the inner "solid" layer, where bacteria is sparce [41, 42]. Only mucin-degrading bacteria like *Akkermansia muciniphila* reach to the inner solid layer. Some pathogens like *Helicobacter pylori*, *Salmonella*, *Yersinia*, *Campylobacter*, etc. can also reach the inner mucus layer [43, 44]. All these factors play an important role in the establishment and the distribution of the gut microbiota.

The initially colonized microbiome has relatively few bacterial species. But during the initial phase of life, bacterial diversity increases in the microbiota. This may be because of the constant exposure of the baby to the environment. The gradual increase in the length of the GI tract can also provide a new niche for the bacteria to colonize. The bacterial diversity also depends on the diet as the introduction of a more plant-based diet increases the proportion of the Firmicutes [45]. Though lifestyle, illness, puberty, and other variable factors affect the microbiome, family members tend to have similar microbiomes with shared bacterial strains [35]. Thus, during the first year of life, the microbiome proceeds through a very variable phase. A distinct composition resembling the "adult microbiome composition" is established once an adult diet is established after weaning [35]. Once established, the gut microbiome composition seems to remain stable for a long time, possibly lifelong [46].

3. Maintain the flora!—on how any alterations could be disastrous

Biologically, the gut microbiome is very essential for the normal functioning of the human body. This complex ecosystem is responsible for many critical functions like (1) metabolism and energy regulation [47]—up to 10% of our daily consumed calories are provided by the microbes who break down complex plant-derived carbohydrates into short-chain fatty acids (SCFA), the main energy source of the enterocytes. From this perspective, alterations in the gut microbiome can contribute to obesity [48, 49] and consequently type II diabetes [50]; (2) immune system activation [51–53]—the colonic mucosal immune system plays a dual role and in that it must tolerate the gut microbiome and at the same time react against pathogenic organisms. This homeostasis is achieved by the intricate interplay between the microbiome and the host; (3) colonization resistance—physiologically colonized body surfaces are intrinsically protected from pathogen colonization. It is the intricate interplay between the above mentioned three major functions of the gut microbiota that brings about the physiological healthy state of the host.

Colonization resistance is the native ability of the host to suppress the invasion by exogenous microorganisms [54]. The concept of colonization resistance originated from the studies of Dubos in 1965 who demonstrated that indigenous gut microbiota neutralize colonization by a potential pathogen [55]. Slightly earlier, it was noted that loss of obligate anaerobic bacterial population in the lower intestinal tract correlated with infection, suggesting that the commensal anaerobic organisms were providing colonization resistance [56–59]. At the time, colonization resistance was thought to result from microbe-mediated inhibition. We now know that the multiple mechanisms like microbiota-mediated activation of host immune responses are also involved. Colonization resistance provides broad protection against bacteria, virus, and other categories of pathogens [60]. On the other hand pathogenic microorganisms can out compete commensal microorganisms, subvert the immune response and invade the epithelia. For example, some pathogens can cause inflammation in the gut and utilize the consequent nutrient-rich inflammatory environment to outgrow other Proteobacteria. However, in a healthy intestine, the gut microbiota maintains the stiff colonization resistance by three mechanisms (1) directly inhibiting or killing the invading organism, (2) maintaining a protective musical barrier, and (3) stimulating a strong immune response that can neutralize a pathogen.

3.1 Direct inhibition

Bacteria produce many bioactive molecules, such as antimicrobial peptides, bacteriocins, etc., to selectively kill or inhibit the growth of competing bacteria [61]. These bioactive molecules are the primary source of antibiotics in the pharmaceutical industry [62].

3.2 Barrier maintenance

Gut microbiota regulates the strength of the intestinal barrier and sequesters themselves within the intestine. For example, the mucus layer is an important deterrent for many pathogenic microorganisms to reach the underlying epithelial cells. Mucus production is enhanced when a germ-free mice epithelium is exposed to some bacterial products [63], which means that an intact microbiota is essential to maintain the required thickness of the mucosal layer to keep pathogenic microorganism at bay. Diet can also influence the thickness of the mucosal layer. An assessment of intestinal microbiota localization with immunofluorescence shows that the absence of microbiota-accessible carbohydrates in the diet resulted in a thinner mucosal layer, thus exposing the underlying epithelial cells to pathogenic organisms [64]. The thinning of the mucosal layer made mouse susceptible to colitis.

3.3 Immune maturation and inflammation

A healthy microbiota is essential for a healthy immune system. Almost one and half decades ago, it was observed that microbial products secreted from the microbiota induced the colonic immune system by activating anti-inflammatory cells and cytokines. In 2005, a polysaccharide from *Bacteroides fragilis*, an important member of the gut microbiota, was shown to be important in the cellular and physical maturation of a developing immune system [51]. Perhaps, the most immunologically characterized bacterial metabolite synthesized by the microbiota is the Short Chain Fatty Acid (SCFA). In 2009, it was shown that SCFA directly bind G-protein-coupled receptor (GPR43) and activated immune responses [65]. Butyrate is the most characterized SCFA. Butyrate was shown to induce the differentiation of colonic regulatory T cells (Treg) cells in mice. A comparative NMR-based metabolome analysis showed that the concentration luminal butyrate correlated with the number of Treg cells in the colon [52]. Treg cells expressing transcription factor Foxp3 are also important in regulating intestinal inflammation. It was also found that SCFA plays an important role in regulating the function and the size of the colonic Treg pool [53].

Microbes can also directly activate the colonic immune system. Segmented filamentous bacterium (SFB) from the microbiota was shown to adhere tightly to epithelial cells of the terminal ileum with Th17 cells, and this adherence correlated with the induction of inflammatory/antimicrobial defense genes [66]. More recently, bacteria in human feces were subjected to selection based on their potential to induce anti-inflammatory T regulatory cells. It was found that bacteria belonging to cluster XIVa clostridial group induced anti-inflammatory T regulatory cells along with bacteroides species [67, 68]. Gut microbiota can also activate the expression of bacterial C-type lectins in intestinal epithelial cells. The lectin, RegIIIγ, is essential to create a 50-μm clearance zone between the gut microbiota and small intestinal epithelial cells. Abrogation of the RegIIIγ synthesis increased the proximity of gut microbiota to the epithelial cells [69]. This shows that microbiota-activated lectin synthesis can directly act to suppress bacterial activity. In addition, gut microbiota can also enhance systemic antiviral activity [70]. Therefore, it is very important to maintain a healthy microbiota to drive efficient pro-inflammatory and anti-inflammatory immune responses in the host.

Simple alterations to the gut microbiota can often lead to very unhealthy consequences. For example, in the esophagus, the composition of the microbiome is heavily dependent on the microbes originating from the oral cavity and is dominated by *Streptococcus, Prevotella, Veillonella*, and *Fusobacterium* [71–73]. Any alteration to the microbiota composition could lead to inflammation and tumorigenesis. Such altered microbiota compositions were consistent with conditions like gastroesophageal reflux disease (GERD), Barrett's esophagus (BE), and adenocarcinoma of the gastro-esophageal (GE) junction. Here, *Streptococcus* were found to be depleted while *Veillonella, Prevotella, Campylobacter, Fusobacterium, Haemophilus*, and *Neisseria* were enriched [74, 75]. Certain taxa present in the oral cavity like *Campylobacter concisus* and *Campylobacter rectus* were found to be enriched in the diseased mucosa-associated with GERD and BE [76, 77]. Similarly, for eosinophilic esophagitis (EoE), increased levels of *Neisseria, Corynebacterium*, and *Haemophilus* are reported [78].

The most important stomach associated bacterium is *H. pylori*. *H. pylori* has symbiotically co-evolved with humans and therefore are highly adapted to humans [79]. Early life time infection of *H. pylori* is beneficial for humans because it significantly lowers the risk of asthma in later years [80]. This beneficial association is brought about by the immune system modulation by the bacterium due to the high induction of regulatory T cells. The bacterium therefore qualifies for the position of a pathobiont -host determines whether the bacteria remains as a harmless symbiont or becomes pathogenic in nature. In a diseased condition of the host, the bacterium outcompetes the normal microbiota in numbers and becomes the most dominant pathogen.

Sampling the fecal material represents the colonic microbial population. However, sampling the small intestine is difficult because it is accessible only by invasive sampling. The small intestine is populated by distinct microbial communities that are less diverse and are dominated by *Veillonella, Streptococcus, Lactobacillus*, and *Clostridium* [81–83]. In the small intestine, alterations in the microbiome are associated with celiac disease (CeD). Gut microbiota is able to differentially degrade gluten. In CeD patients, there is an over growth of an opportunistic pathogen *Pseudomonas aeruginosa* producing a elastase called LasB. This enzyme degrades gluten and releases peptides that translocate the intestinal barrier, triggering a T-cell response [84]. A small-intestine-associated autoimmune disease where microbiome plays an important role is graft versus host disease (GvHD)— caused by the activation of T cells where host cells are recognized as antigens cause autoimmune attacks in the GI tract, liver, lung, and skin [85]. Germ-free mice had less propensity to develop GvHD—this led to the thought that microbiome could play an important role [86–88]. Loss of microbiome diversity and consequent butyrate deprivation pushed cells to apoptosis bearing hallmark histological signs associated with GvHD. An overabundance of *Enterococcus* (*E. faecium* and *E. faecalis*) was observed in patients with GvHD associated with hematopoietic stem cell transfer confirming the association of GvHD with alteration in the microbiome diversity [89].

3.4 Antibiotic-associated colitis

Antibiotics considered as "wonder drugs" were implemented into therapy years before and have saved millions of lives. Even though antibiotics can reduce morbidity and mortality associated with bacterial illness, no antibiotic is pathogen selective. The application of antibiotics lead to collateral damage of accompanying microorganisms in a population, for example in a microbiota. Studies investigating the impact of antibiotics on microbiota confirm that antibiotic treatment increases the susceptibility of an individual to bacterial pathogens by compromising colonization resistance [90–93].

The observation that antibiotic therapy reduced colonization resistance making the host susceptible to bacterial infections was observed very early in the literature [56–59]. Gut microbial compositional analysis of an antibiotic-treated mice showed the expansion of γ-proteobacteria and enterococci, suggesting that gut microbiota somehow suppressed the expansion of oxygen-tolerant species [94, 95]. A study on healthy volunteers treated for a week or less with antibiotics reported persistent effects on their bacterial flora that included a loss of biodiversity on the gut flora, insurgence of antibiotic resistance strains, and upregulation of antibiotic resistance genes [96]. Antibiotic treatment can also induce long-term defects in the microbiota. For example, a single dose of clindamycin induced long-term susceptibility to *Clostridium difficile* infection [92]. A prior treatment with antibiotics not only disturbed the gut microbiota enabling the expansion of pathogenic commensals but also helped exogenic bacterial pathogens to establish inside the gut. When antibiotic-treated mice was infected with vancomycin-resistant *Enterococci* (VRE), the bacteria displaced the whole normal microbiota of the small and large intestine. In the clinical setting, this initial domination by the VRE preceded the bloodstream infections in patients undergoing hematopoietic stem cell transplant [91].

Microbiota establishes itself very early in the life cycle of every human, and this development is very crucial for a healthy lifestyle [97]. So, administration of antibiotics in the early stages of life predisposes the individual to diseases in late infancy or adulthood, particularly allergic or metabolic syndromes [28]. Antibiotic exposed prenatal mice resulted in exacerbated asthma following intranasal challenge with ovalbumin [98]. This case is true in children who are administered with antibiotics in the first year of life and may develop asthma during sixth or the seventh year [99]. Early use of marcolids in Finnish children led to the development of asthma and increased BMI associated with a dysbiotic gut microbiota [100]. Effects of antibiotic administration in early life are not limited to development of asthma alone but also to obesity. A low dose of penicillin delivered at birth transiently shifted the microbiota, and this transient shift induced sustained effects in body composition, leading to obesity [101]. All these reports emphasize the detrimental microbiota-associated effects of antibiotics and their implications in health.

Clostridium difficile is perhaps the most characterized pathogen associated with antibiotic associated colitis [102]. With >25,000 annual cases worldwide, *C. difficile* colitis is almost always associated with prior antibiotic use. The suspicion that microbiota-mediated colonization resistance resisted *C. difficile* in the gut was finally proven in 2013 [103]. 16S rDNA sequencing alone could distinguish between *C. difficile*-associated diarrhea and *C. difficile*-negative diarrhea [104]. Antibiotic treatment reduces secondary bile salt production making the host susceptible to *C. difficile* infection [105, 106]. Apart from *C. difficile*, *Klebsiella oxytoca* also caused antibiotic-associated hemorrhagic colitis (AAHC)—a patchy hemorrhagic colitis usually observed after penicillin therapy typically dominating the right colon. Here, the pathogen is intrinsically resistant to β-lactams and the production of enterotoxin tilivalline can lead to intestinal epithelial apoptosis and colitis [107, 108]. Antibiotic-treated mice had impaired innate and adaptive antiviral immune response, and when the mucosa was exposed to influenza virus, the clearance was substantially delayed. On the other hand, these mice had severe bronchiole epithelial degeneration and increased host mortality when exposed to influenza. This is due to the macrophages from an antibiotic-treated mice had decreased expression of genes associated with antiviral immunity [70].

3.5 Inflammatory bowel disease (IBD)

IBD perhaps is the first diseased condition where alterations in microbiota are studied most extensively. IBD is a term mainly used to describe two disease conditions—Crohn's disease and ulcerative colitis. Here, intestinal cells play an important role in integrating the interactions among intestinal microbiota, mucosal immune system, and environmental factors [109]. It was observed very early that IBD conditions had a genetic component—there was a 10-fold increase in risk if related closely to the patient [110]. Genome-wide association studies (GWAS) reported many genetic factors that are associated with IBD [111]. As more GWAS based studies began identifying genetic factors associated with IBD, it was soon noted that some IBD genetic factors were also associated with other disease conditions like diabetes [112]. Curiously, GWAS and meta-analysis identified considerable overlap between susceptibility loci for IBD and mycobacterial infections [113]. The genetic associations notwithstanding, alterations in the gut microbiome of IBD patients have always been an interesting topic for microbiome researchers. The most significant alteration in the composition of the gut microbiome associated with IBD is the reduction in the abundance of the protective bacterium *Faecalibacterium prausnitzii* [114]. However, patterns of gut microbiota dysbiosis was not consistent across different studies. In a large cohort study involving more than 400 pediatric cases, multiple samples obtained from multiple locations of the GI tract before and after the onset of Crohn's disease were analyzed. Increased abundance of *Enterobacteriaceae*, *Pasteurellaceae*, *Veillonellaceae*, and *Fusobacteriaceae* and decreased abundance of *Erysipelotrichales*, *Bacteroidales*, and *Clostridiales* were found to be strongly consistent with the diseased condition. Oddly enough, there seems to be prevalence of oral bacteria in IBD and Crohn's disease patients. For example, the prevalence of oral and stomach-associated *C. concisus* was very high in both diseased conditions [115]. Furthermore, another Gram-negative oral bacteria *Fusobacterium nucleatum* was found to be abundant in Crohn's disease [116]. *F. nucleatum* was shown to be highly proinflammatory and protumorigenic [117–119]. The bacterium can activate the epithelial cell proliferation and induce a protomeric microenvironment, while inactivating the immunological tumor surveillance.

3.6 Colorectal cancers (CRC)

CRC is the fourth leading causes of death causing cancer and is the third important cause of malignancy. The CRC incidence is growing fast worldwide in low and middle east countries and is expected to increase by 60% by 2030 worldwide [120]. The transformation from a healthy epithelial cell to a malignant cell requires three steps: (1) induction of oncogenic mutations within Lgr5+ intestinal stem cells, (2) altered β-catenin/Wnt signaling, and (3) proinflammatory cascades such as TNFα-NFκB and IL16-STAT3 catalyzing CRC development (Garret 2015 EN). Initially, there was increasing evidence about the role of bacteria in CRC. Bacteria such as *Fusobacterium nucleatum, E. coli*, and *Bacteroides fragilis* were shown to be associated with CRC [117, 121]. *F. nucleatum* was first shown to be highly enriched in tumors [117, 122]. The bacterium produces the FadA antigen, a ligand of E-cadherin in the intestinal epithelial cells that activate the β-catenin pathway leading to uncontrolled cell growth [119]. Furthermore, *F. nucleatum* is shown to be overrepresented in the colonic mucosa in the cases where the CRC relapses postchemotherapy. This was shown to be an interplay of intricate mechanisms including TLRs, miRNAs, and autophagy induction [123]. Some strains of *E. coli* harbor the polyketide synthase (pks) island encoding colibactin, capable of inducing DNA damage and mutation in epithelial cells [121]. A metagenome-wide association study on stools collected from patients with advanced adenomas, CRC, and healthy controls identified that certain *Bacteroides* species (*B. dorei*, *B. vulgaris, B. massiliensis*) and *E. coli* were overrepresented in the microbiome. Similarly, *Parvimonas, Bilophila wadsworthia, Fusobacterium nucleatum*, and *Alistipes* spp. were also overrepresented, suggesting that the gut microbiome signature can be used for early diagnosis and treatment [124].

4. The therapeutic potential of the gut microbiota

Humans have used live bacteria, particularly probiotic bacteria, for therapeutic purposes from time immemorial. We have seen some examples in earlier sections of this chapter. Perhaps, the best example of using live bacteria to cure infectious disease comes from antibiotic-associated CDI illness. *Clostridium scindens*, an obligate anaerobic bacterial species that inhabits the colon, has the rare ability to convert primary bile salts to secondary bile salts and is highly associated with resistance to *C. difficile* colitis [125]. Administration of *C. scindens* to susceptible mice resuscitated the secondary bile salt deficiency and rendered the animal more resistant to CDI. *C. scindens* and *C. difficile* have a negative correlation-could be the reason for *C. difficile* resistance in a healthy human gut microbiota [105]. However, the clinical benefit of using a single bacteria is limited. This is because, as we have seen earlier, many of the disorders are caused by a dysbiotic microbiota. Since a microbiota is very diverse in nature, resuscitation of a healthy gut microbiota cannot be achieved by the administration of a single bacterium. The concept of "putting back the bugs" was demonstrated in 1993 by using a combination of probiotic strains to cure chronic constipations and IBS [126]. Even with CDI, a cocktail of 10 gut commensal bacteria including obligate anaerobes could effect a cure [127]. Since then, many experiments have shown that by replenishing the healthy composition of a normal microbiota, many disease conditions can be controlled. Therefore targeting gut microbiota has gathered much attention and many options are currently being evaluated to achieve this goal of re-establishing the healthy gut microbiota to regain health—leading to the concept of fecal microbiota transplant (FMT).

FMT is the procedure where fecal matter is collected from a tested donor, diluted in an isotonic solution, strained, and transplanted into the patient using colonoscopy, endoscopy, sigmoidoscopy, or enema. The history of using stool of healthy donors to treat human diseases dates back to the fourth century in China, during the Dong Jin dynasty (AD 300–400 years) [128]. Fecal suspensions or "yellow soup" was used to treat serious disorders such as food poisoning, febrile disease, typhoid fever, etc., becoming the first record of the utilization of human feces to treat human diseases. There are striking similarities between the earlier yellow soup and modern day FMT technology—(1) the inoculum originated from human fecal matter, (2) administration route is digestive tract, and (3) the fecal matter re-establishes the microbiota thereby treating the disease. This long tradition might be the reason why FMT is so well accepted in China [129]. In Europe, the first report of using fecal enema to treat pseudomembranous colitis came in 1958 [130]. Currently, FMT stands in the threshold of becoming a great technology to cure many disorders considered incurable in the past.

4.1 In treating diseases associated with gut microbiota-associated dysbiosis

CDI perhaps was the first condition in which a treatment was attempted using FMT. In 1983, it was shown that by re-establishing the healthy gut microbiota using FMT, mitigation of CDI can be achieved (Schwan 1983 EN). Severe CDI cases can lead to intensive care admission, sepsis, toxic megacolon, and can prove fatal. Colectomy is the standard method of treatment, but the mortality rate is 50%. In a study involving 29 patients who underwent FMT plus vancomycin for severe CDI cases, 62% of the patients were cured in a single FMT, while 38% needed multiple FMTs. Taken together, FMT was highly efficient for CDI infections [131]. The primary and secondary cure rates with FMT using fresh fecal sample to cure CDI is 91 and 98% [132]. FMT from frozen fecal sample also gave similar efficacies in treating CDI [133, 134]. By 2013, FMT was made officially the treatment strategy for CDI [103, 135]. Many pharmaceutical firms are actively working to bring easily consumable CDI-targeted drugs based on FMT. A defined microbial ecosystem therapeutics (MET-1 or RePOOPulate) was developed to cure recurrent CDI [136, 137]. The closest enema-based drug that is awaiting clinical approval is RBX2660, which depends upon the microbial suspension provided from the donor and is formulated for therapeutic delivery. With positive results in phase 2, the drug is currently in phase 3.

Similar to CDI, IBD is also a dysbiotic-associated disease where FMT is a potential therapy. However, in IBD, the use of FMT is a bit complicated and less efficient than in CDI. Early studies using FMT to treat IBD showed very promising result with good microbiota remission reported over long-term follow up [138]. With years, the outcomes started to differ depending upon sample size, treatment approaches, and study designs [139]. Even within IBD patients, remission rates were different. Crohn's disease had a higher remission of 61%, while ulcerative colitis patients had a remission rate of 22%. It is clear that the FMT treatment for IBD is complicated by numerous factors like differences in treatment regimens, stool preparation/formulation, and dosing frequencies. Varied levels of dysbiosis and difference in the microbiota composition between donor and patient also complicate FMT treatments. However, it was reported that FMT with intensive doses and multiple donors induced clinical remission and endoscopic improvement in ulcerative colitis patients, and this treatment had distinctive improvements in the microbiota composition [140]. It was also shown that a second FMT 3 months past the first one greatly improved the efficacy and safety in treating IBD with FMT [141, 142]. Here, the patients received FMT repeatedly in 3 month intervals—in a procedure called step-up FMT. The efficacy of the procedure increased at each step and was best suggested for patients with refractory IBD and immune-related diseases [143, 144]. There are currently 27 ongoing clinical trials using FMT targeting IBD with two additional trials on children with IBD [145].

Cancers like colorectal cancers that are associated with a dysbiotic microbiome opening the possibility for a therapeutic intervention using FMT. It was shown that bacteria like *Enterococcus hirae* and *Barnesiella intestinihominis* strengthen cyclophosphamide-induced therapeutic immunomodulatory effects in cancer [146]. This has been highlighted very recently with evidence that microbiome influences with body's ability to respond to antibody therapy for cancers [147, 148]. A correlation was observed between commensal microbial composition and clinical response to anti-PD-L1 therapy through abundance of bacterial species like *Bifidobacterium longum*, *Collinsella aerofaciens*, and *Enterococcus faecium* [149]. When fecal matter from responding patients were transplanted to germ-free mice, the animals were noted with stronger tumor control, augmented T cell responses, and better efficacy [150]. Gut microbiota could also affect anticancer responses with CTLA-4 [151]. The effects of radiation in gut microbiota and the clinical implications of a modified microbial balance postradiotherapy are now being investigated [152]. The microbiota can be modified to improve its efficacy and reduce the toxic burden of these treatments [153]. FMT can be used to reduce the radiation-induced toxicity and the increase the survival rate in irradiated mice. Here, the WBCs, GI tract function, and intestinal epithelial cell integrity were improved [154]. The research advances notwithstanding, therapeutic approaches associated with FMT is still in its nascent stage. However, considerable progress made in this area of research indicate that the application of FMT based therapy to mitigate mortality associated with diseases like cancer is a near possibility.

FMT is also showing great promise in patients undergoing hematopoietic stem cell transplantation surgery. Administration of a series of prophylactic antibiotics during surgery can result in the loss of microbial gut diversity and antibiotic resistant strains like *Streptococcus viridans*, *Enterococcus faecium*, and other Enterobacteriaceae can expand their population in the gut. This loss of microbial diversity during stem cell transplantation is associated with marked increase in mortality [91, 155, 156]. Restoration of a healthy microbiota by eliminating the dominant pathogenic microorganisms therefore becomes very important strategy from a therapeutic point of view. FMT involving a consortium of obligate anaerobic commensal bacteria containing especially *Barnesiella* is shown to eliminate *E. faecium* in mice [157], opening up a new therapeutic approach for stem cell transplant patients.

4.2 Collection, preparation, and delivery of FMT samples

Collection and preservation of the stool samples carry the primary importance in FMT. Freshly collected feces can either be immediately used, lyophilized, or cryopreserved. The efficacy of FMT in treating CDI using fresh or frozen feces varied but not significantly [158]. The cure rate was 100% in patients receiving fresh feces, 83% for the lyophilized group, and 78% for patients receiving frozen feces. But the efficacy was more pronounced in treating IBD, and this was demonstrated to be caused due to loss of bacteria in frozen feces [143]. The laboratory preparation methods of FMT is also critical for the success of FMT. Recent studies have reported that some preparation methods can stress the living microbial cells affecting the efficacy of FMT [159] emphasizing the need for extreme care. For example, *Faecalibacterium prausnitzii* is affected when the fecal sample is exposed to oxygen. Currently, the preparation methods can be classified into "rough filtration" (RF), "filtration plus centrifugation" (FPC), and "microfiltration plus centrifugation" (MPC) [141, 142]. Manual preparation methods takes about 6 hours to complete [160]. With the introduction of automated systems and close cooperation between laboratory scientists and clinicians, the time period of preparation from "defecation to freezing" has been shortened to 1 hour [160]— has effectively increased the efficacy of FMT when tested against IBD patients [143]. Current FMT delivery technologies include delivery of the microbiota to upper, mid, and the lower gut [161]. Oral intake of capsular microbiota delivers it to the upper gut [134, 162]. A suspension of microbiota infusion can be transferred to the small intestine beyond the second duodenal segment through endoscopy [163], nasojejunal tube [143], mid-gut transendoscopic enteral tubing (TET) [164], and percutaneous endoscopic gastro-jejunostomy (PEG-J) [161]. The TET procedure for microbiota transplant is considered very successful [164]. Delivery of microbiota to the lower gut could be through colonoscopy, enema, distal ileum stoma, colostomy, and colonic TET [161]. Colonic TET is recommended for patients needing frequent FMT.

Several groups are developing stool products that can be packaged, transported, commercialized, and easily administered by physicians or consumed by patients. These products range from basic (frozen or freeze-dried stool) to more advanced products like capsules of synthetic stool grown in culture and assembled. The most basic products, from stool banks like OpenBiome and Advancing Bio, provide hospitals with screened frozen material ready for clinical use. More advanced are products like RBX2660, a cryopreserved filtered microbiota derived from stool of selected donors and administered via an enema system. The most advanced is a lyophilized powder that can be reconstituted by rectal infusions developed by CIPAC Therapeutics.

4.3 Precision microbiome reconstitution

The lack of regulatory protocol and stiff resistance from clinicians treating chronically ill patients has dampened efforts to introduce FMT as a viable therapy. This led to the development of the concept of "precision microbiome reconstitution," where a single bacterium can be used to restore colonization resistance in *C. difficile* patients [105]—providing a more targeted approach where a consortia of specific bacterial strains are identified to treat a particular diseased condition, and this will enable greater specificity and quality control. In germ-free mice, a murine isolate belonging to the family *Lachnospiraceae* partially restored colonization resistance against *C. difficile* [165]. An elaborate study using mouse models, clinical studies, metagenomic analysis, and mathematical modeling identified *C. scindens* as an intestinal bacterium associated with resistance to *C. difficile*. *C. scindens* produces growth inhibitory or spore germination inhibitory secondary bile acids to inhibit *C. difficile*. Furthermore, colonic induction of anti-inflammatory T regulatory cells can be used to develop immunity against dysbiotic conditions. A community of 17 strains including *C. scindens* induced the development of anti-inflammatory T regulatory cells, and this reduced colitis [67]. They also identified that the concentration of short-chain fatty acids increased upon the colonization of these 17 isolates. The fact that short-chain fatty acids modulated a Treg cell response suggested a common pathway by which different microbes modulated an induction of Treg cells. This opportunity was utilized to identify many more strains mostly belonging to bacteroides that are capable to induce an immune response that can restore colonization resistance from a dysbiotic condition [68]. However, even though a single strain may be able to resist a single organism of interest, a community of organisms reflecting the diversity of microbiota might be needed to restore baseline colonization resistance. This specific targeted approach is used by pharmaceutical firms to develop targeted drugs—for example, Seres Therapeutics is developing SER-109—comprising bacterial spores enriched and purified from healthy stool and packaged into capsules. The product can restructure a dysbiotic gut to a healthy microbiome. Vedanta Biosciences are identifying and developing bacterial strains that can suppress chronic gut inflammation. Similarly, a microbial assemblage derived from stool and grown in culture called RePOOPulate has been developed to treat CDI infections.

4.4 The importance of SAFE FMT

Safety of the patient should be of prime importance when an FMT procedure is considered, especially if the patient is having a poor immune status [166, 167]. Middle gut FMT procedures can cause vomiting and aspiration [168]. The nasojejunal tube could put the patient at high risk of aspiration and should be conducted with anesthesia [143]. There is enough evidence that the long-term safety of the patient should be considered as well. Generally, a tested donor fecal sample is used for FMT. However, this carries the disadvantage that unwanted or potentially pathogenic bacterial phenotypes maybe carried from donors to recipients. A particular case was reported where the patient developed new onset obesity after obtaining a stool sample from a heterologous donor [169]. Using the patient's own stool sample can avoid the problems associated with donor stool samples. Here, a fecal sample of the patient is banked in the hospital before any procedure that requires antibiotic treatment. The banked sample may provide the vital resource to avoid hospital-acquired infections and to replenish the patient's own microbiota. Preservation of the patient's own or donor feces pose a second challenge [170]. There are reports that fecal matter from patients with colon cancer promoted tumorigenesis in germ-free and carcinogenic mice. Potential cardiometabolic, autoimmune, and neurological disease also have been discussed. All these points to the tough screening and regulations are needed before a donor is selected for fecal sample prior FMT.

However, recent reports suggest that FMT is gaining wide acceptance among patients. A survey showed that among patients of Crohn's disease who received FMT, 56% showed satisfactory clinical efficacy, 74% showed willingness for a second FMT, and 89% expressed willingness to recommend FMT to other patients [171]. Also, the cost efficacy of FMT has been demonstrated worldwide [172–176, 177]. FMT is still very far from being implemented into routine therapy. The technique needs to undergo rigorous process of standardization before the therapy becomes applied in daily practice. Nevertheless the importance of gut microbiota in maintenance of a healthy lifestyle is demonstrated without doubt. In future therapeutic approaches including antibiotic therapy should take into consideration the impact it has on the gut microbiota and the clinicians should be mindful of the impact of the devastating secondary effects of these therapeutic approaches on the patient.

Author details

Shabarinath Srikumar* and Séamus Fanning
UCD-Centre for Food Safety, School of Public Health, Physiotherapy and Sports
Science, University College Dublin, Ireland

*Address all correspondence to: srikumar.shabarinath@ucd.ie

IntechOpen

References

[1] Human Microbiome Project C. A framework for human microbiome research. Nature. 2012;**486**(7402):215-221

[2] Qin J, Li R, Raes J, Arumugam M, Burgdorf KS, Manichanh C, et al. A human gut microbial gene catalogue established by metagenomic sequencing. Nature. 2010;**464**(7285):59-65

[3] Halwachs B, Madhusudhan N, Krause R, Nilsson RH, Moissl-Eichinger C, Hogenauer C, et al. Critical issues in mycobiota analysis. Frontiers in Microbiology. 2017;**8**:180

[4] Sender R, Fuchs S, Milo R. Are we really vastly outnumbered? Revisiting the ratio of bacterial to host cells in humans. Cell. 2016;**164**(3):337-340

[5] Neish AS. Microbes in gastrointestinal health and disease. Gastroenterology. 2009;**136**(1):65-80

[6] Human Microbiome Project C. Structure, function and diversity of the healthy human microbiome. Nature. 2012;**486**(7402):207-214

[7] Donaldson GP, Lee SM, Mazmanian SK. Gut biogeography of the bacterial microbiota. Nature Reviews. Microbiology. 2016;**14**(1):20-32

[8] Duncan SH, Louis P, Flint HJ. Cultivable bacterial diversity from the human colon. Letters in Applied Microbiology. 2007;**44**(4):343-350

[9] O'Hara AM, Shanahan F. The gut flora as a forgotten organ. EMBO Reports. 2006;**7**(7):688-693

[10] Flint HJ, Scott KP, Duncan SH, Louis P, Forano E. Microbial degradation of complex carbohydrates in the gut. Gut Microbes. 2012;**3**(4):289-306

[11] LeBlanc JG, Milani C, de Giori GS, Sesma F, van Sinderen D, Ventura M. Bacteria as vitamin suppliers to their host: A gut microbiota perspective. Current Opinion in Biotechnology. 2013;**24**(2):160-168

[12] Duncan SH, Scott KP, Ramsay AG, Harmsen HJ, Welling GW, Stewart CS, et al. Effects of alternative dietary substrates on competition between human colonic bacteria in an anaerobic fermentor system. Applied and Environmental Microbiology. 2003;**69**(2):1136-1142

[13] Round JL, Mazmanian SK. The gut microbiota shapes intestinal immune responses during health and disease. Nature Reviews. Immunology. 2009;**9**(5):313-323

[14] Sommer F, Backhed F. The gut microbiota—Masters of host development and physiology. Nature Reviews. Microbiology. 2013;**11**(4):227-238

[15] Kelly CJ, Zheng L, Campbell EL, Saeedi B, Scholz CC, Bayless AJ, et al. Crosstalk between microbiota-derived short-chain fatty acids and intestinal epithelial HIF augments tissue barrier function. Cell Host & Microbe. 2015;**17**(5):662-671

[16] Reinhardt C, Bergentall M, Greiner TU, Schaffner F, Ostergren-Lunden G, Petersen LC, et al. Tissue factor and PAR1 promote microbiota-induced intestinal vascular remodelling. Nature. 2012;**483**(7391):627-631

[17] Luna RA, Foster JA. Gut brain axis: Diet microbiota interactions and implications for modulation of anxiety and depression. Current Opinion in Biotechnology. 2015;**32**:35-41

[18] Mayer EA, Tillisch K, Gupta A. Gut/brain axis and the microbiota.

The Journal of Clinical Investigation. 2015;**125**(3):926-938

[19] Mu C, Yang Y, Zhu W. Gut microbiota: The brain peacekeeper. Frontiers in Microbiology. 2016;7:345

[20] Collins SM, Surette M, Bercik P. The interplay between the intestinal microbiota and the brain. Nature Reviews. Microbiology. 2012;**10**(11):735-742

[21] Carmody RN, Gerber GK, Luevano JM Jr, Gatti DM, Somes L, Svenson KL, et al. Diet dominates host genotype in shaping the murine gut microbiota. Cell Host & Microbe. 2015;**17**(1):72-84

[22] Zarrinpar A, Chaix A, Yooseph S, Panda S. Diet and feeding pattern affect the diurnal dynamics of the gut microbiome. Cell Metabolism. 2014;**20**(6):1006-1017

[23] Thaiss CA, Zeevi D, Levy M, Zilberman-Schapira G, Suez J, Tengeler AC, et al. Transkingdom control of microbiota diurnal oscillations promotes metabolic homeostasis. Cell. 2014;**159**(3):514-529

[24] DeGruttola AK, Low D, Mizoguchi A, Mizoguchi E. Current understanding of dysbiosis in disease in human and animal models. Inflammatory Bowel Diseases. 2016;**22**(5):1137-1150

[25] Hyman RW, Fukushima M, Diamond L, Kumm J, Giudice LC, Davis RW. Microbes on the human vaginal epithelium. Proceedings of the National Academy of Sciences of the United States of America. 2005;**102**(22):7952-7957

[26] Zhou X, Brown CJ, Abdo Z, Davis CC, Hansmann MA, Joyce P, et al. Differences in the composition of vaginal microbial communities found in healthy Caucasian and black women. The ISME Journal. 2007;**1**(2):121-133

[27] Ravel J, Gajer P, Abdo Z, Schneider GM, Koenig SS, McCulle SL, et al. Vaginal microbiome of reproductive-age women. Proceedings of the National Academy of Sciences of the United States of America. 2011;**108**(Suppl 1): 4680-4687

[28] Dominguez-Bello MG, Costello EK, Contreras M, Magris M, Hidalgo G, Fierer N, et al. Delivery mode shapes the acquisition and structure of the initial microbiota across multiple body habitats in newborns. Proceedings of the National Academy of Sciences of the United States of America. 2010;**107**(26):11971-11975

[29] Costello EK, Lauber CL, Hamady M, Fierer N, Gordon JI, Knight R. Bacterial community variation in human body habitats across space and time. Science. 2009;**326**(5960):1694-1697

[30] Fanaro S, Chierici R, Guerrini P, Vigi V. Intestinal microflora in early infancy: Composition and development. Acta Paediatrica. Supplement. 2003;**91**(441):48-55

[31] Favier CF, Vaughan EE, De Vos WM, Akkermans AD. Molecular monitoring of succession of bacterial communities in human neonates. Applied and Environmental Microbiology. 2002;**68**(1):219-226

[32] Palmer C, Bik EM, DiGiulio DB, Relman DA, Brown PO. Development of the human infant intestinal microbiota. PLoS Biology. 2007;**5**(7):e177

[33] Mackie RI, Sghir A, Gaskins HR. Developmental microbial ecology of the neonatal gastrointestinal tract. The American Journal of Clinical Nutrition. 1999;**69**(5):1035S-1045S

[34] Coppa GV, Zampini L, Galeazzi T, Gabrielli O. Prebiotics in human milk: A review. Digestive and Liver Disease. 2006;**38**(Suppl 2):S291-S294

[35] Turnbaugh PJ, Hamady M, Yatsunenko T, Cantarel BL, Duncan A, Ley RE, et al. A core gut microbiome in obese and lean twins. Nature. 2009;**457**(7228):480-484

[36] Biasucci G, Benenati B, Morelli L, Bessi E, Boehm G. Cesarean delivery may affect the early biodiversity of intestinal bacteria. The Journal of Nutrition. 2008;**138**(9):1796S-1800S

[37] Biasucci G, Rubini M, Riboni S, Morelli L, Bessi E, Retetangos C. Mode of delivery affects the bacterial community in the newborn gut. Early Human Development. 2010;**86**(Suppl 1): 13-15

[38] Penders J, Thijs C, van den Brandt PA, Kummeling I, Snijders B, Stelma F, et al. Gut microbiota composition and development of atopic manifestations in infancy: The KOALA Birth Cohort Study. Gut. 2007;**56**(5):661-667

[39] Bager P, Wohlfahrt J, Westergaard T. Caesarean delivery and risk of atopy and allergic disease: Meta-analyses. Clinical and Experimental Allergy. 2008;**38**(4):634-642

[40] Albenberg L, Esipova TV, Judge CP, Bittinger K, Chen J, Laughlin A, et al. Correlation between intraluminal oxygen gradient and radial partitioning of intestinal microbiota. Gastroenterology. 2014;**147**(5):1055-1063 e1058

[41] Johansson ME, Larsson JM, Hansson GC. The two mucus layers of colon are organized by the MUC2 mucin, whereas the outer layer is a legislator of host-microbial interactions. Proceedings of the National Academy of Sciences of the United States of America. 2011;**108**(Suppl 1):4659-4665

[42] Tropini C, Earle KA, Huang KC, Sonnenburg JL. The gut microbiome: Connecting spatial organization to function. Cell Host & Microbe. 2017;**21**(4):433-442

[43] Berry D, Stecher B, Schintlmeister A, Reichert J, Brugiroux S, Wild B, et al. Host-compound foraging by intestinal microbiota revealed by single-cell stable isotope probing. Proceedings of the National Academy of Sciences of the United States of America. 2013;**110**(12):4720-4725

[44] Pedron T, Mulet C, Dauga C, Frangeul L, Chervaux C, Grompone G, et al. A crypt-specific core microbiota resides in the mouse colon. MBio. 2012;**3**(3):e00116-12

[45] Koenig JE, Spor A, Scalfone N, Fricker AD, Stombaugh J, Knight R, et al. Succession of microbial consortia in the developing infant gut microbiome. Proceedings of the National Academy of Sciences of the United States of America. 2011;**108**(Suppl 1):4578-4585

[46] Backhed F, Roswall J, Peng Y, Feng Q, Jia H, Kovatcheva-Datchary P, et al. Dynamics and stabilization of the human gut microbiome during the first year of life. Cell Host & Microbe. 2015;**17**(5):690-703

[47] Nieuwdorp M, Gilijamse PW, Pai N, Kaplan LM. Role of the microbiome in energy regulation and metabolism. Gastroenterology. 2014;**146**(6):1525-1533

[48] Turnbaugh PJ, Ley RE, Mahowald MA, Magrini V, Mardis ER, Gordon JI. An obesity-associated gut microbiome with increased capacity for energy harvest. Nature. 2006;**444**(7122):1027-1031

[49] Ley RE, Turnbaugh PJ, Klein S, Gordon JI. Microbial ecology: Human gut microbes associated with obesity. Nature. 2006;**444**(7122):1022-1023

[50] Sonnenburg JL, Backhed F. Diet-microbiota interactions as moderators of human metabolism. Nature. 2016;**535**(7610):56-64

[51] Mazmanian SK, Liu CH, Tzianabos AO, Kasper DL. An immunomodulatory molecule of symbiotic bacteria directs maturation of the host immune system. Cell. 2005;**122**(1):107-118

[52] Furusawa Y, Obata Y, Fukuda S, Endo TA, Nakato G, Takahashi D, et al. Commensal microbe-derived butyrate induces the differentiation of colonic regulatory T cells. Nature. 2013;**504**(7480):446-450

[53] Smith PM, Howitt MR, Panikov N, Michaud M, Gallini CA, Bohlooly YM, et al. The microbial metabolites, short-chain fatty acids, regulate colonic Treg cell homeostasis. Science. 2013;**341**(6145):569-573

[54] Stecher B, Maier L, Hardt WD. 'Blooming' in the gut: How dysbiosis might contribute to pathogen evolution. Nature Reviews. Microbiology. 2013;**11**(4):277-284

[55] Mushin R, Dubos R. Colonization of the mouse intestine with *Escherichia coli*. The Journal of Experimental Medicine. 1965;**122**(4):745-757

[56] Bohnhoff M, Drake BL, Miller CP. Effect of streptomycin on susceptibility of intestinal tract to experimental Salmonella infection. Proceedings of the Society for Experimental Biology and Medicine. 1954;**86**(1):132-137

[57] Bohnhoff M, Miller CP. Enhanced susceptibility to Salmonella infection in streptomycin-treated mice. The Journal of Infectious Diseases. 1962;**111**:117-127

[58] Freter R. The fatal enteric cholera infection in the guinea pig, achieved by inhibition of normal enteric flora. The Journal of Infectious Diseases. 1955;**97**(1):57-65

[59] Hentges DJ, Freter R. In vivo and in vitro antagonism of intestinal bacteria against Shigella flexneri.

I. Correlation between various tests. The Journal of Infectious Diseases. 1962;**110**:30-37

[60] Ichinohe T, Pang IK, Kumamoto Y, Peaper DR, Ho JH, Murray TS, et al. Microbiota regulates immune defense against respiratory tract influenza A virus infection. Proceedings of the National Academy of Sciences of the United States of America. 2011;**108**(13):5354-5359

[61] Kommineni S, Bretl DJ, Lam V, Chakraborty R, Hayward M, Simpson P, et al. Bacteriocin production augments niche competition by enterococci in the mammalian gastrointestinal tract. Nature. 2015;**526**(7575):719-722

[62] Milshteyn A, Schneider JS, Brady SF. Mining the metabiome: Identifying novel natural products from microbial communities. Chemistry & Biology. 2014;**21**(9):1211-1223

[63] Petersson J, Schreiber O, Hansson GC, Gendler SJ, Velcich A, Lundberg JO, et al. Importance and regulation of the colonic mucus barrier in a mouse model of colitis. American Journal of Physiology. Gastrointestinal and Liver Physiology. 2011;**300**(2):G327-G333

[64] Earle KA, Billings G, Sigal M, Lichtman JS, Hansson GC, Elias JE, et al. Quantitative imaging of gut microbiota spatial organization. Cell Host & Microbe. 2015;**18**(4):478-488

[65] Maslowski KM, Vieira AT, Ng A, Kranich J, Sierro F, Yu D, et al. Regulation of inflammatory responses by gut microbiota and chemoattractant receptor GPR43. Nature. 2009;**461**(7268):1282-1286

[66] Ivanov II, Atarashi K, Manel N, Brodie EL, Shima T, Karaoz U, et al. Induction of intestinal Th17 cells by segmented filamentous bacteria. Cell. 2009;**139**(3):485-498

[67] Atarashi K, Tanoue T, Oshima K, Suda W, Nagano Y, Nishikawa H, et al. Treg induction by a rationally selected mixture of Clostridia strains from the human microbiota. Nature. 2013;**500**(7461):232-236

[68] Faith JJ, Ahern PP, Ridaura VK, Cheng J, Gordon JI. Identifying gut microbe-host phenotype relationships using combinatorial communities in gnotobiotic mice. Science Translational Medicine. 2014;**6**(220):220ra211

[69] Vaishnava S, Yamamoto M, Severson KM, Ruhn KA, Yu X, Koren O, et al. The antibacterial lectin RegIIIgamma promotes the spatial segregation of microbiota and host in the intestine. Science. 2011;**334**(6053):255-258

[70] Abt MC, Osborne LC, Monticelli LA, Doering TA, Alenghat T, Sonnenberg GF, et al. Commensal bacteria calibrate the activation threshold of innate antiviral immunity. Immunity. 2012;**37**(1):158-170

[71] Nardone G, Compare D, Rocco A. A microbiota-centric view of diseases of the upper gastrointestinal tract. Lancet Gastroenterology & Hepatology. 2017;**2**(4):298-312

[72] Hunt RH, Yaghoobi M. The esophageal and gastric microbiome in health and disease. Gastroenterology Clinics of North America. 2017;**46**(1):121-141

[73] Di Pilato V, Freschi G, Ringressi MN, Pallecchi L, Rossolini GM, Bechi P. The esophageal microbiota in health and disease. Annals of the New York Academy of Sciences. 2016;**1381**(1):21-33

[74] Yang L, Lu X, Nossa CW, Francois F, Peek RM, Pei Z. Inflammation and intestinal metaplasia of the distal esophagus are associated with alterations in the microbiome. Gastroenterology. 2009;**137**(2):588-597

[75] Liu N, Ando T, Ishiguro K, Maeda O, Watanabe O, Funasaka K, et al. Characterization of bacterial biota in the distal esophagus of Japanese patients with reflux esophagitis and Barrett's esophagus. BMC Infectious Diseases. 2013;**13**:130

[76] Blackett KL, Siddhi SS, Cleary S, Steed H, Miller MH, Macfarlane S, et al. Oesophageal bacterial biofilm changes in gastro-oesophageal reflux disease, Barrett's and oesophageal carcinoma: Association or causality? Alimentary Pharmacology & Therapeutics. 2013;**37**(11):1084-1092

[77] Macfarlane S, Furrie E, Macfarlane GT, Dillon JF. Microbial colonization of the upper gastrointestinal tract in patients with Barrett's esophagus. Clinical Infectious Diseases. 2007;**45**(1):29-38

[78] Benitez AJ, Hoffmann C, Muir AB, Dods KK, Spergel JM, Bushman FD, et al. Inflammation-associated microbiota in pediatric eosinophilic esophagitis. Microbiome. 2015;**3**:23

[79] Falush D, Wirth T, Linz B, Pritchard JK, Stephens M, Kidd M, et al. Traces of human migrations in *Helicobacter pylori* populations. Science. 2003;**299**(5612):1582-1585

[80] Arnold IC, Dehzad N, Reuter S, Martin H, Becher B, Taube C, et al. *Helicobacter pylori* infection prevents allergic asthma in mouse models through the induction of regulatory T cells. The Journal of Clinical Investigation. 2011;**121**(8):3088-3093

[81] Wang M, Ahrne S, Jeppsson B, Molin G. Comparison of bacterial diversity along the human intestinal tract by direct cloning and sequencing of 16S rRNA genes. FEMS Microbiology Ecology. 2005;**54**(2):219-231

[82] Hartman AL, Lough DM, Barupal DK, Fiehn O, Fishbein T, Zasloff M,

et al. Human gut microbiome adopts an alternative state following small bowel transplantation. Proceedings of the National Academy of Sciences of the United States of America. 2009;**106**(40):17187-17192

[83] Booijink CC, El-Aidy S, Rajilic-Stojanovic M, Heilig HG, Troost FJ, Smidt H, et al. High temporal and inter-individual variation detected in the human ileal microbiota. Environmental Microbiology. 2010;**12**(12):3213-3227

[84] Caminero A, Galipeau HJ, McCarville JL, Johnston CW, Bernier SP, Russell AK, et al. Duodenal bacteria from patients with celiac disease and healthy subjects distinctly affect gluten breakdown and immunogenicity. Gastroenterology. 2016;**151**(4):670-683

[85] Staffas A, Burgos da Silva M, van den Brink MR. The intestinal microbiota in allogeneic hematopoietic cell transplant and graft-versus-host disease. Blood. 2017;**129**(8):927-933

[86] van Bekkum DW, Roodenburg J, Heidt PJ, van der Waaij D. Mitigation of secondary disease of allogeneic mouse radiation chimeras by modification of the intestinal microflora. Journal of the National Cancer Institute. 1974;**52**(2):401-404

[87] Jones JM, Wilson R, Bealmear PM. Mortality and gross pathology of secondary disease in germfree mouse radiation chimeras. Radiation Research. 1971;**45**(3):577-588

[88] Taur Y, Jenq RR, Perales MA, Littmann ER, Morjaria S, Ling L, et al. The effects of intestinal tract bacterial diversity on mortality following allogeneic hematopoietic stem cell transplantation. Blood. 2014;**124**(7):1174-1182

[89] Holler E, Butzhammer P, Schmid K, Hundsrucker C, Koestler J, Peter K, et al. Metagenomic analysis of the stool microbiome in patients receiving allogeneic stem cell transplantation: Loss of diversity is associated with use of systemic antibiotics and more pronounced in gastrointestinal graft-versus-host disease. Biology of Blood and Marrow Transplantation. 2014;**20**(5):640-645

[90] Dethlefsen L, McFall-Ngai M, Relman DA. An ecological and evolutionary perspective on human-microbe mutualism and disease. Nature. 2007;**449**(7164):811-818

[91] Ubeda C, Taur Y, Jenq RR, Equinda MJ, Son T, Samstein M, et al. Vancomycin-resistant Enterococcus domination of intestinal microbiota is enabled by antibiotic treatment in mice and precedes bloodstream invasion in humans. The Journal of Clinical Investigation. 2010;**120**(12):4332-4341

[92] Buffie CG, Jarchum I, Equinda M, Lipuma L, Gobourne A, Viale A, et al. Profound alterations of intestinal microbiota following a single dose of clindamycin results in sustained susceptibility to *Clostridium difficile*-induced colitis. Infection and Immunity. 2012;**80**(1):62-73

[93] Buffie CG, Pamer EG. Microbiota-mediated colonization resistance against intestinal pathogens. Nature Reviews. Immunology. 2013;**13**(11):790-801

[94] Vollaard EJ, Clasener HA, Janssen AJ. Decontamination of the bowel by intravenous administration of pefloxacin. The Journal of Antimicrobial Chemotherapy. 1990;**26**(6):847-852

[95] Vollaard EJ, Clasener HA, van Griethuysen AJ, Janssen AJ, Sanders-Reijmers AJ. Influence of amoxicillin, erythromycin and roxithromycin on colonization resistance and on appearance of secondary colonization in healthy volunteers. The Journal of Antimicrobial Chemotherapy. 1987;**20**(Suppl B):131-138

[96] Jernberg C, Lofmark S, Edlund C, Jansson JK. Long-term ecological impacts of antibiotic administration on the human intestinal microbiota. The ISME Journal. 2007;**1**(1):56-66

[97] Dominguez-Bello MG, Blaser MJ, Ley RE, Knight R. Development of the human gastrointestinal microbiota and insights from high-throughput sequencing. Gastroenterology. 2011;**140**(6):1713-1719

[98] Russell SL, Gold MJ, Hartmann M, Willing BP, Thorson L, Wlodarska M, et al. Early life antibiotic-driven changes in microbiota enhance susceptibility to allergic asthma. EMBO Reports. 2012;**13**(5):440-447

[99] Risnes KR, Belanger K, Murk W, Bracken MB. Antibiotic exposure by 6 months and asthma and allergy at 6 years: Findings in a cohort of 1,401 US children. American Journal of Epidemiology. 2011;**173**(3):310-318

[100] Korpela K, Salonen A, Virta LJ, Kekkonen RA, Forslund K, Bork P, et al. Intestinal microbiome is related to lifetime antibiotic use in Finnish pre-school children. Nature Communications. 2016;**7**:10410

[101] Cox LM, Yamanishi S, Sohn J, Alekseyenko AV, Leung JM, Cho I, et al. Altering the intestinal microbiota during a critical developmental window has lasting metabolic consequences. Cell. 2014;**158**(4):705-721

[102] Britton RA, Young VB. Role of the intestinal microbiota in resistance to colonization by *Clostridium difficile*. Gastroenterology. 2014;**146**(6):1547-1553

[103] van Nood E, Vrieze A, Nieuwdorp M, Fuentes S, Zoetendal EG, de Vos WM, et al. Duodenal infusion of donor feces for recurrent *Clostridium difficile*. The New England Journal of Medicine. 2013;**368**(5):407-415

[104] Schubert AM, Rogers MA, Ring C, Mogle J, Petrosino JP, Young VB, et al. Microbiome data distinguish patients with *Clostridium difficile* infection and non-*C. difficile*-associated diarrhea from healthy controls. MBio. 2014;**5**(3):e01021-e01014

[105] Buffie CG, Bucci V, Stein RR, McKenney PT, Ling L, Gobourne A, et al. Precision microbiome reconstitution restores bile acid mediated resistance to *Clostridium difficile*. Nature. 2015;**517**(7533):205-208

[106] Theriot CM, Koenigsknecht MJ, Carlson PE Jr, Hatton GE, Nelson AM, Li B, et al. Antibiotic-induced shifts in the mouse gut microbiome and metabolome increase susceptibility to *Clostridium difficile* infection. Nature Communications. 2014;**5**:3114

[107] Hogenauer C, Langner C, Beubler E, Lippe IT, Schicho R, Gorkiewicz G, et al. Klebsiella oxytoca as a causative organism of antibiotic-associated hemorrhagic colitis. The New England Journal of Medicine. 2006;**355**(23):2418-2426

[108] Schneditz G, Rentner J, Roier S, Pletz J, Herzog KA, Bucker R, et al. Enterotoxicity of a nonribosomal peptide causes antibiotic-associated colitis. Proceedings of the National Academy of Sciences of the United States of America. 2014;**111**(36):13181-13186

[109] Kaser A, Zeissig S, Blumberg RS. Inflammatory bowel disease. Annual Review of Immunology. 2010;**28**:573-621

[110] Orholm M, Munkholm P, Langholz E, Nielsen OH, Sorensen TI, Binder V. Familial occurrence of inflammatory bowel disease. The New England Journal of Medicine. 1991;**324**(2):84-88

[111] Barrett JC, Hansoul S, Nicolae DL, Cho JH, Duerr RH, Rioux JD, et al.

Genome-wide association defines more than 30 distinct susceptibility loci for Crohn's disease. Nature Genetics. 2008;**40**(8):955-962

[112] Lees CW, Barrett JC, Parkes M, Satsangi J. New IBD genetics: Common pathways with other diseases. Gut. 2011;**60**(12):1739-1753

[113] Jostins L, Ripke S, Weersma RK, Duerr RH, McGovern DP, Hui KY, et al. Host-microbe interactions have shaped the genetic architecture of inflammatory bowel disease. Nature. 2012;**491**(7422):119-124

[114] Becker C, Neurath MF, Wirtz S. The intestinal microbiota in inflammatory bowel disease. ILAR Journal. 2015;**56**(2):192-204

[115] Castano-Rodriguez N, Kaakoush NO, Lee WS, Mitchell HM. Dual role of Helicobacter and Campylobacter species in IBD: A systematic review and meta-analysis. Gut. 2017;**66**(2):235-249

[116] Gevers D, Kugathasan S, Denson LA, Vazquez-Baeza Y, Van Treuren W, Ren B, et al. The treatment-naive microbiome in new-onset Crohn's disease. Cell Host & Microbe. 2014;**15**(3):382-392

[117] Kostic AD, Chun E, Robertson L, Glickman JN, Gallini CA, Michaud M, et al. Fusobacterium nucleatum potentiates intestinal tumorigenesis and modulates the tumor-immune microenvironment. Cell Host & Microbe. 2013;**14**(2):207-215

[118] Gur C, Ibrahim Y, Isaacson B, Yamin R, Abed J, Gamliel M, et al. Binding of the Fap2 protein of Fusobacterium nucleatum to human inhibitory receptor TIGIT protects tumors from immune cell attack. Immunity. 2015;**42**(2):344-355

[119] Rubinstein MR, Wang X, Liu W, Hao Y, Cai G, Han YW. Fusobacterium nucleatum promotes colorectal carcinogenesis by modulating E-cadherin/beta-catenin signaling via its FadA adhesin. Cell Host & Microbe. 2013;**14**(2):195-206

[120] Arnold M, Sierra MS, Laversanne M, Soerjomataram I, Jemal A, Bray F. Global patterns and trends in colorectal cancer incidence and mortality. Gut. 2017;**66**(4):683-691

[121] Arthur JC, Perez-Chanona E, Muhlbauer M, Tomkovich S, Uronis JM, Fan TJ, et al. Intestinal inflammation targets cancer-inducing activity of the microbiota. Science. 2012;**338**(6103):120-123

[122] Castellarin M, Warren RL, Freeman JD, Dreolini L, Krzywinski M, Strauss J, et al. Fusobacterium nucleatum infection is prevalent in human colorectal carcinoma. Genome Research. 2012;**22**(2):299-306

[123] Yu T, Guo F, Yu Y, Sun T, Ma D, Han J, et al. Fusobacterium nucleatum promotes chemoresistance to colorectal cancer by modulating autophagy. Cell. 2017;**170**(3):548-563 e516

[124] Feng Q, Liang S, Jia H, Stadlmayr A, Tang L, Lan Z, et al. Gut microbiome development along the colorectal adenoma-carcinoma sequence. Nature Communications. 2015;**6**:6528

[125] Lawley TD, Clare S, Walker AW, Stares MD, Connor TR, Raisen C, et al. Targeted restoration of the intestinal microbiota with a simple, defined bacteriotherapy resolves relapsing *Clostridium difficile* disease in mice. PLoS Pathogens. 2012;**8**(10):e1002995

[126] Andrews PJ, Borody TJ. "Putting back the bugs": Bacterial treatment relieves chronic constipation and symptoms of irritable bowel syndrome. The Medical Journal of Australia. 1993;**159**(9):633-634

[127] Tvede M, Rask-Madsen J. Bacteriotherapy for chronic relapsing *Clostridium difficile* diarrhoea in six patients. Lancet. 1989;1(8648):1156-1160

[128] Zhang F, Luo W, Shi Y, Fan Z, Ji G. Should we standardize the 1,700-year-old fecal microbiota transplantation? American Journal of Gastroenterology. 2012;**107**(11):1755; author reply p 1755-1756

[129] Ren RR, Sun G, Yang YS, Peng LH, Wang SF, Shi XH, et al. Chinese physicians' perceptions of fecal microbiota transplantation. World Journal of Gastroenterology. 2016;**22**(19):4757-4765

[130] Eiseman B, Silen W, Bascom GS, Kauvar AJ. Fecal enema as an adjunct in the treatment of pseudomembranous enterocolitis. Surgery. 1958;**44**(5):854-859

[131] Fischer M, Sipe BW, Rogers NA, Cook GK, Robb BW, Vuppalanchi R, et al. Faecal microbiota transplantation plus selected use of vancomycin for severe-complicated *Clostridium difficile* infection: Description of a protocol with high success rate. Alimentary Pharmacology & Therapeutics. 2015;**42**(4):470-476

[132] Brandt LJ, Aroniadis OC, Mellow M, Kanatzar A, Kelly C, Park T, et al. Long-term follow-up of colonoscopic fecal microbiota transplant for recurrent *Clostridium difficile* infection. The American Journal of Gastroenterology. 2012;**107**(7):1079-1087

[133] Hamilton MJ, Weingarden AR, Sadowsky MJ, Khoruts A. Standardized frozen preparation for transplantation of fecal microbiota for recurrent *Clostridium difficile* infection. The American Journal of Gastroenterology. 2012;**107**(5):761-767

[134] Lee CH, Steiner T, Petrof EO, Smieja M, Roscoe D, Nematallah A, et al. Frozen vs fresh fecal microbiota transplantation and clinical resolution of diarrhea in patients with recurrent *Clostridium difficile* infection: A randomized clinical trial. JAMA. 2016;**315**(2):142-149

[135] Surawicz CM, Brandt LJ, Binion DG, Ananthakrishnan AN, Curry SR, Gilligan PH, et al. Guidelines for diagnosis, treatment, and prevention of *Clostridium difficile* infections. The American Journal of Gastroenterology. 2013;**108**(4):478-498; quiz 499

[136] Petrof EO, Gloor GB, Vanner SJ, Weese SJ, Carter D, Daigneault MC, et al. Stool substitute transplant therapy for the eradication of *Clostridium difficile* infection: 'RePOOPulating' the gut. Microbiome. 2013;**1**(1):3

[137] Martz SL, Guzman-Rodriguez M, He SM, Noordhof C, Hurlbut DJ, Gloor GB, et al. A human gut ecosystem protects against *C. difficile* disease by targeting TcdA. Journal of Gastroenterology. 2017;**52**(4):452-465

[138] Bennet JD, Brinkman M. Treatment of ulcerative colitis by implantation of normal colonic flora. Lancet. 1989;1(8630):164

[139] Kelly CR, Kahn S, Kashyap P, Laine L, Rubin D, Atreja A, et al. Update on fecal microbiota transplantation 2015: Indications, methodologies, mechanisms, and outlook. Gastroenterology. 2015;**149**(1):223-237

[140] Paramsothy S, Kamm MA, Kaakoush NO, Walsh AJ, van den Bogaerde J, Samuel D, et al. Multidonor intensive faecal microbiota transplantation for active ulcerative colitis: A randomised placebo-controlled trial. Lancet. 2017;**389**(10075):1218-1228

[141] He Z, Li P, Zhu J, Cui B, Xu L, Xiang J, et al. Multiple fresh fecal microbiota transplants induces and

maintains clinical remission in Crohn's disease complicated with inflammatory mass. Scientific Reports. 2017;7(1):4753

[142] He Z, Cui BT, Zhang T, Li P, Long CY, Ji GZ, et al. Fecal microbiota transplantation cured epilepsy in a case with Crohn's disease: The first report. World Journal of Gastroenterology. 2017;23(19):3565-3568

[143] Cui B, Feng Q, Wang H, Wang M, Peng Z, Li P, et al. Fecal microbiota transplantation through mid-gut for refractory Crohn's disease: Safety, feasibility, and efficacy trial results. Journal of Gastroenterology and Hepatology. 2015;30(1):51-58

[144] Cui B, Li P, Xu L, Peng Z, Xiang J, He Z, et al. Step-up fecal microbiota transplantation (FMT) strategy. Gut Microbes. 2016;7(4):323-328

[145] Cho JA, Chinnapen DJF. Targeting friend and foe: Emerging therapeutics in the age of gut microbiome and disease. Journal of Microbiology. 2018;56(3):183-188

[146] Daillere R, Vetizou M, Waldschmitt N, Yamazaki T, Isnard C, Poirier-Colame V, et al. *Enterococcus hirae* and *Barnesiella intestinihominis* facilitate cyclophosphamide-induced therapeutic immunomodulatory effects. Immunity. 2016;45(4):931-943

[147] Gopalakrishnan V, Spencer CN, Nezi L, Reuben A, Andrews MC, Karpinets TV, et al. Gut microbiome modulates response to anti-PD-1 immunotherapy in melanoma patients. Science. 2018;359(6371):97-103

[148] Routy B, Le Chatelier E, Derosa L, Duong CPM, Alou MT, Daillere R, et al. Gut microbiome influences efficacy of PD-1-based immunotherapy against epithelial tumors. Science. 2018;359(6371):91-97

[149] Matson V, Fessler J, Bao R, Chongsuwat T, Zha Y, Alegre ML, et al. The commensal microbiome is associated with anti-PD-1 efficacy in metastatic melanoma patients. Science. 2018;359(6371):104-108

[150] Gopalakrishnan V, Helmink BA, Spencer CN, Reuben A, Wargo JA. The influence of the gut microbiome on cancer, immunity, and cancer immunotherapy. Cancer Cell. 2018;33(4):570-580

[151] Vetizou M, Pitt JM, Daillere R, Lepage P, Waldschmitt N, Flament C, et al. Anticancer immunotherapy by CTLA-4 blockade relies on the gut microbiota. Science. 2015;350(6264):1079-1084

[152] Ferreira MR, Muls A, Dearnaley DP, Andreyev HJ. Microbiota and radiation-induced bowel toxicity: Lessons from inflammatory bowel disease for the radiation oncologist. The Lancet Oncology. 2014;15(3):e139-e147

[153] Alexander JL, Wilson ID, Teare J, Marchesi JR, Nicholson JK, Kinross JM. Gut microbiota modulation of chemotherapy efficacy and toxicity. Nature Reviews. Gastroenterology & Hepatology. 2017;14(6):356-365

[154] Cui M, Xiao H, Li Y, Zhou L, Zhao S, Luo D, et al. Faecal microbiota transplantation protects against radiation-induced toxicity. EMBO Molecular Medicine. 2017;9(4):448-461

[155] Taur Y, Xavier JB, Lipuma L, Ubeda C, Goldberg J, Gobourne A, et al. Intestinal domination and the risk of bacteremia in patients undergoing allogeneic hematopoietic stem cell transplantation. Clinical Infectious Diseases. 2012;55(7):905-914

[156] Taur Y, Pamer EG. Harnessing microbiota to kill a pathogen: Fixing the microbiota to treat *Clostridium difficile* infections. Nature Medicine. 2014;20(3):246-247

[157] Ubeda C, Bucci V, Caballero S, Djukovic A, Toussaint NC, Equinda M, et al. Intestinal microbiota containing Barnesiella species cures vancomycin-resistant *Enterococcus faecium* colonization. Infection and Immunity. 2013;**81**(3):965-973

[158] Jiang ZD, Ajami NJ, Petrosino JF, Jun G, Hanis CL, Shah M, et al. Randomised clinical trial: Faecal microbiota transplantation for recurrent *Clostridum difficile* infection—Fresh, or frozen, or lyophilised microbiota from a small pool of healthy donors delivered by colonoscopy. Alimentary Pharmacology & Therapeutics. 2017;**45**(7):899-908

[159] Chu ND, Smith MB, Perrotta AR, Kassam Z, Alm EJ. Profiling living bacteria informs preparation of fecal microbiota transplantations. PLoS One. 2017;**12**(1):e0170922

[160] Cammarota G, Ianiro G, Tilg H, Rajilic-Stojanovic M, Kump P, Satokari R, et al. European consensus conference on faecal microbiota transplantation in clinical practice. Gut. 2017;**66**(4):569-580

[161] Peng Z, Xiang J, He Z, Zhang T, Xu L, Cui B, et al. Colonic transendoscopic enteral tubing: A novel way of transplanting fecal microbiota. Endoscopy International Open. 2016;**4**(6):E610-E613

[162] Youngster I, Russell GH, Pindar C, Ziv-Baran T, Sauk J, Hohmann EL. Oral, capsulized, frozen fecal microbiota transplantation for relapsing *Clostridium difficile* infection. JAMA. 2014;**312**(17):1772-1778

[163] Zhang F, Amateau SK, Khashab MA, Okolo PI 3rd. Mid-gut stents. Current Opinion in Gastroenterology. 2012;**28**(5):451-460

[164] Long C, Yu Y, Cui B, Jagessar SAR, Zhang J, Ji G, et al. A novel quick transendoscopic enteral tubing in mid-gut: Technique and training with video. BMC Gastroenterology. 2018;**18**(1):37

[165] Reeves AE, Koenigsknecht MJ, Bergin IL, Young VB. Suppression of *Clostridium difficile* in the gastrointestinal tracts of germfree mice inoculated with a murine isolate from the family Lachnospiraceae. Infection and Immunity. 2012;**80**(11):3786-3794

[166] Fischer M, Kao D, Mehta SR, Martin T, Dimitry J, Keshteli AH, et al. Predictors of early failure after fecal microbiota transplantation for the therapy of *Clostridium difficile* infection: A multicenter study. The American Journal of Gastroenterology. 2016;**111**(7):1024-1031

[167] Fischer M, Kao D, Kelly C, Kuchipudi A, Jafri SM, Blumenkehl M, et al. Fecal microbiota transplantation is safe and efficacious for recurrent or refractory *Clostridium difficile* infection in patients with inflammatory bowel disease. Inflammatory Bowel Diseases. 2016;**22**(10):2402-2409

[168] Gweon TG, Kim J, Lim CH, Park JM, Lee DG, Lee IS, et al. Fecal microbiota transplantation using upper gastrointestinal tract for the treatment of refractory or severe complicated clostridium difficile infection in elderly patients in poor medical condition: The first study in an Asian country. Gastroenterology Research and Practice. 2016;**2016**:2687605

[169] Alang N, Kelly CR. Weight gain after fecal microbiota transplantation. Open Forum Infectious Diseases. 2015;**2**(1):ofv004

[170] Hale VL, Tan CL, Niu K, Yang Y, Cui D, Zhao H, et al. Effects of field conditions on fecal microbiota. Journal of Microbiological Methods. 2016;**130**:180-188

[171] Xu L, Zhang T, Cui B, He Z, Xiang J, Long C, et al. Clinical efficacy maintains patients' positive attitudes toward fecal microbiota transplantation. Medicine (Baltimore). 2016;**95**(30):e4055

[172] Konijeti GG, Sauk J, Shrime MG, Gupta M, Ananthakrishnan AN. Cost-effectiveness of competing strategies for management of recurrent Clostridium difficile infection: A decision analysis. Clinical Infectious Diseases. 2014;**58**(11):1507-1514

[173] Varier RU, Biltaji E, Smith KJ, Roberts MS, Kyle Jensen M, LaFleur J, et al. Cost-effectiveness analysis of fecal microbiota transplantation for recurrent *Clostridium difficile* infection. Infection Control and Hospital Epidemiology. 2015;**36**(4):438-444

[174] Waye A, Atkins K, Kao D. Cost averted with timely fecal microbiota transplantation in the management of recurrent *Clostridium difficile* infection in Alberta, Canada. Journal of Clinical Gastroenterology. 2016;**50**(9):747-753

[175] Merlo G, Graves N, Brain D, Connelly LB. Economic evaluation of fecal microbiota transplantation for the treatment of recurrent *Clostridium difficile* infection in Australia. Journal of Gastroenterology and Hepatology. 2016;**31**(12):1927-1932

[176] Baro E, Galperine T, Denies F, Lannoy D, Lenne X, Odou P, et al. Cost-effectiveness analysis of five competing strategies for the management of multiple recurrent community-onset *Clostridium difficile* infection in France. PLoS One. 2017;**12**(1):e0170258

[177] Zhang T, Xiang J, Cui B, He Z, Li P, Chen H, et al. Cost-effectiveness analysis of fecal microbiota transplantation for inflammatory bowel disease. Oncotarget. 2017;**8**(51):88894-88903

Section 3

Microbes in Health and Diseases

Chapter 3

The Role of Leather Microbes in Human Health

Richard O. Oruko, John O. Odiyo and Joshua N. Edokpayi

Abstract

Leather tanned from raw hides and skins have been used to cover and protect the human body since early man. The skin of an animal carries thousands of microbes. Some are beneficial and protect the animal while others are pathogenic and cause diseases. Some microbes have no defined roles in animals. These microbes end up in the human body through contact with the animal skin. In recent years, the human body has been studied as an ecosystem where trillions of microorganisms live as a community called microbiome. Humans need beneficial microbes like *Bacillus subtilis* on the skin surface to stay healthy. Many microbes need the human body to survive. Not many studies have looked into the close link between animal leather and the human microbiome. The assumption is that conventional leather processes inhibit the pathogens on skins from carrying any risk of microbial hazard to the human body. This chapter identifies endemic microbes of "animal skin microbiome" that withstand extreme acidity and alkalinity of leather manufacture and their transmission to humans. Some cause allergic reactions, skin lesion, infections or death to tannery employees with weakened immune systems. This promotes the need to look at leather product microbiome impact on human health.

Keywords: human health, human microbiome, leather-making processes, microbial hazard, pathogens, raw hide and skin and tanned leather

1. General introduction

Skin is the largest organ in the animal's body and acts as the entry point of microbes from the outside world [1, 2]. The diverse population of microbes found in human and animal resides on the skin. About 1000 different species of bacteria, fungi, viruses and other microbes live on the skin. The majority are harmless and even beneficial to human and animal hosts. Microbe colonisation of the skin is normally variable and relies on endogenous host factors, topographical location and exogenous environmental factors [3]. Over a long period of time, microbes, humans and other animals have established complex relationships with each other [2]. For example, to remain healthy, humans and other animals require microbes and many microbes also require specific environments provided by the human and the animal's bodies to sustain their lives. Humans, other animals, and microbes depend on these interactions to grow and stay healthy. Diverse species of microbes reside in different places in and on human and other animals and they are adapted to those conditions and places. Human, animals and their microbial flora form a complex ecosystem whose equilibrium acts as a reliable adaptation system [2]. In realisation of this important complex relationship, the United States government in 2008 launched the human microbiome project. The above-mentioned project emphasised the need for comprehensive characterisation of different body parts for microbial communities of humans [4].

Microbiome research study in animals has lagged behind human research because of lack of investment, towards relating the animal microbiome in human health and disease [4]. "Animal microbiome" is wider in scope than humans, and as such, there is a lot of data specific to each animal species, their body parts, and their products. However, there is a need for animal products microbiome data as that of the human condition, particularly in One Health mindset concept. In this concept, it is necessary to consider the health of the animal and their products, as being closely linked to the health of humans. Globally everybody uses animal skin and leather products in one way or the other in their daily lives. This implies that microbes in them might be interacting with human health either positively or negatively. Microbiome research in this topic is still in nascent's stage and needs to be studied in detail to show the link as this is important, due to the fundamental biology of these invisible microbes in animal skins/leather products and their roles in human health.

2. Microbes reported in animal skins and leather products

Live animals bodies host thousands and thousands of microbes. Some are harmful while others are not. Among the pathogenic microbes are those which can cause diseases in animal and human. These diseases are known as zoonotic diseases. A zoonotic disease or zoonosis is defined as any disease of animals that can be transmitted to people [5]. The first recognised zoonoses with an occupational relationship relevant to the leather industry are those that cause skin lesions and have short incubation periods, such as ringworm infections, cutaneous anthrax and glanders [5]. Anthrax infection among tannery workers has been reported in Bangladesh [6]. The first documented case of anthrax in the United States of America occurred in Florida state in 1974. Cutaneous anthrax occurred due to contact with a goat skin bongo drum bought in Haiti while inhalation anthrax occurred in Scotland in 2006. This happened because of handling contaminated hide drums from West Africa [7]. The most common fungal disease in animal skin is ringworm, also known as *Dermatophytosis*. This is not a worm at all, but a fungus called *Dermatophytes* that grows on the skin. It affects workers who handle raw skins without wearing protective gears in the tanning industry [7].

Other microbes on the live animal skin only cause infection and damage to the skin [8]. It is yet to be known if they can affect humans that handle them. The most important bacterium that causes damage to the skin during the animal's life is *Dermatophilus congolensis*, which occurs as a secondary infection, in bovine demodicosis lesions. *Staphylococcus aureus, Staphylococcus albus*, and *Streptococcus pyogenes* are all reported to be associated with lesions of demodectic mange in sheepskin. *Staphylococcus aureus, Corynebacterium pyogenes, Pseudomonas aeruginosa, Bacillus subtilis*, and *Morexella bovis* have been isolated as secondary infections where bovine demodicosis was found to be present [8]. Some of these microbes have potential to cause pathogens on the host. They are normally transferred from the animal skin to human skin whenever people get into contact with the live animal in the fields or dead animal skin during slaughter. This is common in developing countries where not all skins that reach curing premises and tanneries come from licenced slaughterhouses. Some originate from individual homes; such skins are called "fallen hide/skin". Some come from individual homes located deep in the interior villages, where veterinary services are lacking. This results into skins of a diseased animal, which have not been inspected by a veterinary inspector. The potential to infect the people handling them is always very high if they are affected by the zoonotic disease. This is the first stage of exposure to the workers in the leather manufacture chains and therefore it has become a source of concern about tannery worker health.

As soon as the animal is slaughtered the processes of decay on the flesh side begins. Animal skin undergoes microbiological decay since as an organic material it is a source of food for microbes [8]. Organisms involved in hide and skin putrefaction in slaughterhouses include *Staphylococci* and *Micrococcus* organisms. The majority of *Staphylococci* isolated so far includes *Staphylococcus xylosus, Staphylococcus sciuri, Staphylococcus cohnii, Staphylococcus simulans, Staphylococcus hyicus* and *Staphylococcus epidermidis*. The *Micrococcus* found in this study was *Micrococcus varians* [9]. In one study, 414 micro-organisms from 80 cattle hide and 80 sheep skin swab samples were isolated in Sudan. Out of the above figure, 134 isolates were characterised from fresh and washed cattle hides and sheep skins which included;- *Staphylococcus spp., Micrococcus spp., Corynebacterium spp., Aerococcus homorri, Enterococcus casseliflavus, Aerococcus viridans, Enterococcus faecalis, Gemella haemolysans, Stomatococcus spp., Pseudomonas spp.* and *Escherichia coli*. The samples taken from the slaughterhouse hides and skins were predominately *Staphylococcus spp., Micrococcus spp., Bacillus spp.* and *Corynebacterium spp.* along with *Staphylococcus albus, Streptococcus pyogenes, Pseudomonas aeruginosa, Bacillus subtilis* and *Corynebacterium pyogenes* [10].

From the slaughterhouses, the skins are normally moved to curing premises for preservation before they are delivered to the tannery for processing into leather. Preservation methods used range from sun drying, air drying on frames, salting, brining and chilling. Although these methods stop putrefaction of hides and skins, some microbes still survive and eventually move to the tanning process. Bacteria isolated from hides and skins delivered directly to the tannery without prior treatment include *Staphylococcus spp., Micrococcus spp., Corynebacterium spp., Lactobacillus jensenii, Streptococcus spp., Enterococcus spp., Stomatococcus mucilaginous, Bacillus spp., Aerococcus viridans, Pseudomonas vulgaris biogroup II, Escherichia coli* and *Pseudomonas spp.*

Hides and skins showing signs of putrefaction in the curing premises normally give off an offensive odour and show hair slipping on the grain side. Bacteria involved in putrefaction of those areas have been identified as *Staphylococcus saccharolyticus, Staphylococcus capitis, Staphylococcus hyicus, Micrococcus lylae, Corynebacterium bovis, Cory xerosis, Lactobacillus jensenii, Bacillus cereus, Staphylococcus intermedius, Bacillus amylogliguesta, Staphylococcus saprophyticus, Staphylococcus auricularis, Staphylococcus hominis, Staphylococcus epidermidis, Staphylococcus xylosus, Micrococcus varians* and *Micrococcus lentus*. In general *Staphylococcus spp., Micrococcus spp., Corynebacterium spp., Bacillus spp., E. coli* and *Pseudomonas spp* were found to be common [10]. The following bacteria; *Staphylococcus gallinarum, Dermacoccus nishinomiyaensis, Gardnerella vaginalis* and *Staphylococcus equorum* were isolated from putrefied hides and skins for the first time [10]. *Staphylococcus chromogenes, Staphylococcus xylosus, Staphylococcus kloosii* and *Bacillus mycoides* were found to be growing well in dried hides and skins [11]. The *Staphylococcus spp.* and *Micrococcus spp.* are therefore considered to be part of the normal microflora of cattle hides and sheep skins [11, 12].

Gram-positive and Gram-negative bacteria have also been isolated from goat and sheepskins. Gram-positive bacteria were identified to be 78.7% [13]. The isolated bacteria were identified as *Bacillus cereus, Bacillus subtilis, Bacillus megaterium, Lactobacillus casei, Lactobacillus acidophilus, Lactobacillus fermentum, Micrococcus luteus, Neisseria flavescens, Neisseria sicca, Proteus mirabilis, Proteus spp, Pseudomonas spp, Staphylococcus luteus, Staphylococcus aureus, Staphylococcus epidermis,* and *Streptococcus faecalis*. The writers found out that the Gram-positive Bacilli and Cocci with proteolytic activity are the most responsible for the degradation of goat and sheep skins [13]. These microbes might end up on the bodies of workers in the leather manufacture chain. Their consequences on the health of these tannery workers could be detrimental if they are potentially pathogenic.

Many curing premises use salt to preserve green hides and skins. In the salted cattle hides and sheepskins the following bacteria have been isolated; *Staphylococcus spp, Micrococcus spp., Corynebacterium spp., Enterococcus spp., Stomatococcus mucilaginosus, Bacillus spp., Moraxella bovis, Proteus vulgaris biogroup II, Pseudomonas spp.* and *Escherichia coli* [14]. These bacteria are considered salt-resistant species especially *Staphylococcus, Micrococcus, Corynebacterium, Stomatococcus, Lactobacillus,* and *Bacillus*. The writers consider them halophilic bacteria since they can grow well in salt concentrations of 5–15% [15]. Other reported studies indicate that on a salted raw hide, the proliferation of halophilic bacteria results in the production of a range of pigments giving red and violet spots. From these coloured spots *Micrococcus roseus, Micrococcus luteus* and *Micrococcus morrhuae* have most frequently been isolated [15, 16]. Fungi have also been confirmed to be natural inhabitants of hides/skins. Fungi species can tolerate high NaCI concentrations of 20–30% (w/v) [17]. This is a higher concentration than that tolerated by bacteria. *Aspergillus terreus, Aspergillus niger, Aspergillus fumigatus, Penicillium restrictum, Penicillium citrinum, Altemia spp.* and *Cladosporium spp.* were isolated from salted sheepskins [17]. From the curing premises, the raw hides and skins are taken to tanneries for processing. The first stage of tanning is the beamhouse yard.

In the beamhouse operations, six perforation-causing strains of bacteria have been isolated and identified as belonging to *Bacillus subtilis, Bacillus megaterium, Bacillus anthracoides, Bacillus pumilus* and *Pseudomonas aeruginosa*. They were isolated from soaking water for raw skin in the beam house [18]. An environmental mycological survey carried out at the liming section of the Tannery and Footwear Corporation (TAFCO) at Kanpur, India, in 1985, isolated and characterised 33 fungal species. *Aspergillus spp.* and *Penicillium spp.* were the two predominantly isolated fungal species. The other isolated species were *Alternaria spp., Cephalosporium spp., Chaetomium spp., Cladosporium spp., Cunninghamella spp., CUNularia spp., Drechslera spp., Fusarium spp., Mucor spp., Phoma spp., Rhizopus spp.* and *Trichoderma spp* [18]. The following isolated fungal species from beamhouse have been reported to have potential allergens. They include *Aspergillus flavus, Aspergillus oryzae, Aspergillus sulphureus, Aspergillus sydowii, Aspergillus terreus, Mucor geophila* and *Rhizopus stolonifer* [18]. Various fungal species such as *Penicillium spp., Aspergillus spp., Alternaria spp., Scopulariopsis spp.* and *Cladosporium spp.* have also been isolated from 14 tanneries in Istanbul, Turkey. *Penicillium spp.* was found to be the most commonly isolated fungal species followed by *Aspergillus spp* [19]. The authors, therefore concluded that the allergen from the isolated fungal species may be the reason for the development of respiratory infections in tannery workers thus the need to pay more attention to the skin microbes from leather industries even those which are undergoing processing.

From the beamhouse yard, the leather processing moves to tanyard operation. Here we have chrome-tanned leather (known technically as wet blue) with the formation of red spots which is a frequent phenomenon in the tanned leather. The originators of the red colour on tanned leather have been identified as *Paecilomyces ehrlichii* (=*Penicillium klebanii*), *Penicillium aculeatum, Penicillium purpurogenum* and *Penicillium Roseopurpureum* [20]. The red spots on the wet blue are not limited to one type of leather only, since these fungi attack and cause red colouration even in box sides, horse chevreau, pig-skin splits and goat skins, among others. From tanyard operations, leather processing moves to crust and finishing yard. During drying of finished leathers, moulds may also develop due to favourable humidities and temperatures inside the drying rooms [20]. On the other hand, the biodeterioration becomes visible as spots of various sizes in green, yellow-brown, dark-brown, grey and brown-green shades on the finished leather. Associated with this type of damage, various workers have isolated *Aspergillus ochraceus, Aspergillus wentii, Penicillium rugulosum, Penicillium funiculosum, Penicillium variotii* and *V. glaucum*. They are noted for attacking skin substrates with high grease content, but a far larger range of fungal types than these cause damage during leather drying process.

Major damage on finished leathers is caused by fungi. The types of fungus that are encountered in tanneries are well-known contaminants of leather materials [21]. Those that are frequently isolated includes; *Penicillium chrysogenum, Penicillium luteum, Penicillium brevicompactum, Penicillium decumbens, Penicillium rugulosum, Penicillium aculeatum, Penicillium funiculosum, Aspergillus niger, Aspergillus fumigatus, Aspergillus ochraceus, Aspergillus wentii, Aspergillus < avus-oryzae (group), Mucor mucedo, Rhizopus nigricans, Paecilomyces variotii, S. brevicaulis, V. glaucum* and *Trichoderma viride*. The above mentioned fungi utilise tanning conditions for their growth and development, hence they can even be found on the finished leathers as well as on the surface of vegetable-tanning solutions. In these solutions, they cause fermentation of the tanning agent due to the effect of "tannase" enzymes especially in the production of vegetable-tanned sole leathers. A poor growth of the yeasts *Candida albicans* and the moderate growth of *Staphylococcus aureus* were observed on the finished leather specimen [21]. The reported researches have proved that *Penicillium, Aspergillus*, and *Trichoderma* are the main microbes growing on the wet blue leather [22].

A new kind of bacterial defect, different from well-known bacteria-borne defects (like hair slip, red discolouration, and grain pilling) on the leather has also been identified. It is called the bio-film. A biofilm defect is explained to be composed of a single or multiple species of bacteria, embedded in the polyanionic extracellular polymeric substances which are attached to the surface of leather [23]. Different bacterial and fungal species, for example, the Genus of *Bacillus, Corynebacterium, Clostridium, Staphylococcus, Penicillium, Aspergillus, Paecilomyces, Candida*, and *Cryptococcus* are responsible for destruction and degradation of leather and their products [24, 25]; therefore, these microbes with potential pathogens could pose a real threat to the health of tannery workers and even the population that use leather goods.

Finished leather is normally used to make leather items like the belt, purse, shoes, upholstery and boots, among others. A study carried out around 2015 in Mauritius found that purses used by almost everybody globally could be a potential reservoir for bacteria, in particular, those made out of leather and synthetic materials [26]. In roughly half of the purses sampled in that study, there was only a single type of bacterial growth isolated and identified. In the other half of the samples, there was the identification of mixed growth. In most cases, these microbes are normally carried harmlessly on the skin of most people. It is reported by some authors that infection only occur if a person has a weak immune system or if the skin is wounded, allowing the bacteria to enter the body [26]. Therefore, it is worth noting that even finished leather items are potential sources of pathogenic microbes. Besides that, finished leather products such as footwear may be colonised by fungi and bacteria [27]. The carbon source for bacterial growth is sweat compounds of footwear users and other compounds contained in shoe materials. Footwear, especially those often and intensively used, provides an ideal environment for microbial growth, including pathogenic species, causing athlete's foot (tinea pedis) and bacterial foot infections. This is connected with a favourable temperature and high moisture content inside the shoes, enhancing microbial growth [27]: A poor growth of yeasts *Candida albicans* and moderate growth of *Staphylococcus aureus* was observed under specimens of leather finished without essential oils. However, no growth of *Escherichia coli* was recorded [28], thus microbes in the raw skin go beyond the tanning process and therefore it is relevant to take note of the leather microbiome and their possible effect on human health. This can be done by adding effective fungicides and bacteriocides on processed leather with less effect on human health.

3. Reported cases of beneficial microbes on humans from leather products

Micro-organisms with the symbiotic relationship with the skin occupy a wide range of skin niches and can protect it against invasion by harmful organisms. One such type of bacteria that is known to protect the skin is *Bacillus subtilis*. It produces bacitracin on the skin surface, a toxin that helps it in fighting with other intruding microbes [1, 2]. These skin microflora may also have a role in educating billions of T cells, making them ready to respond to similarly marked pathogen [3]. Most of the time in our lifetime, we share our bodies harmoniously with the 90 trillion or so microbes [29]. By simply taking or applying antibiotics, we could be disturbing the stable ecosystem in our body by killing not only disease-causing micro-organisms but also good bacteria, like *Lactobacillus acidophilus* which protects the body against pathogenic bacteria. A balanced co-existence between microbes and human bodies requires appropriate use of antibiotic and reserving the good role these organisms play in the animal and human health. Some resident microbes are known to protect animals against pathogens. Evidence attributed to this comes mainly from studies performed with germ-free animals, which were found to be extremely sensitive to infection and some died following the administration of a pathogen [30].

Microbes on the skin and other parts of the body have been known to protect it against environmental toxic materials, such as heavy metals, hydrazine, fungal, plant toxins, oxalic acid among others [30]. It is also speculated that changes in temperature, present problem to some animals that cannot use their skin to regulate their body temperature. This regards how to carry out cellular metabolism at both high and low temperatures. Some microbiotas can help solve this problem by providing enzymes optimised for different temperatures. On the other hand, an animal's microbial symbiotic partners may as well play a significant role in helping select the trait of endothermy. The constant high temperature of the surrounding environment speeds up bacterial fermentation by providing rapid and sustained energy input for the host. These benefits become apparent when comparing conventional to germ-free mammals, which sometimes require one-third more food to maintain the same body mass [30]. Some good bacteria inhibit fungal growth in parts of the skins. For, an example in the forearm of a human there are over 100 species of bacteria that keep the skin healthy. On average, it is reported that the skin supports about 1 trillion bacteria species. The most common among them are *Staphylococcus, Streptococcus*, and *Corynebacterium,* which metabolise sweat on skin surface to produce the bad odour. Most of these mentioned bacteria actually help to keep the skin healthy by competing with dangerous pathogens for nutrients and growth space. *Firmicutes* and *Bacteroides* are known to break down carbohydrates and make essential nutrients like vitamins K and B12 for the animal's body development. They also block out harmful bacteria from invading the skin.

Other evidence suggested by different authors, states that commensal skin microbes are necessary and sufficient for the generation of optimal skin immunity. This has been observed from germ-free mice in an experiment. The mice failed to mount an adequate immune response to *Leishmania* disease. Recolonisation of the mice gut with microbes was unable to restore cutaneous immune function to this animal, but exposing the skin of these mice to *S. epidermidis* alone was sufficient to restore the effect or T cell levels and rescue the immune deficiency from total collapse. These observations according to the writer were linked to IL-1 signalling, as germ-free mice showed significant decreases in cutaneous IL-1α production. The evidence adduced here suggests that communication between commensal microbes and skin-resident cells is important for proper tuning of the local inflammatory milieu [1, 2, 30]. The potential impacts of commensal microbiota from leather on the response and development of an effective immune environment on the human skin are still unclear and therefore require further studies.

Fungi are also beneficial partners in symbiosis with the animal's skin [31]. This microbe has the ability to grow on vertebrate animal skins. Some fungi species can attack insects and nematodes in the skin and in the long run play an important role in keeping populations of these animals under control. Insect-attacking fungi are called "*Entomopathogens*," and they include a wide range of fungi in phyla *Ascomycota*, *Zygomycota*, and *Chytridiomycota*. Some of the best-known and most spectacular *Entomopathogens* among them belong to the *Ascomycota* genus *Ophiocordyceps* [31]. Beneficial microbes that are not mentioned here have other roles inside the animal's body. There are also some microbes with unknown roles in the skin of the animals yet they occur there abundantly. Some have been isolated but others are yet to be isolated and cultured. They make the study of leather microbiome necessary.

4. Mechanism of microbes transfer from animal skins and leather products to humans

The human skin might also be affected by the microbes from the animal's skin with which they get into close contact [32]. Previous studies as reported by other authors on European populations have shown that the skin microbial communities of dog owners are closely similar to the microbial communities of their dogs than those of other dogs. The report goes on to confirm that close contact with dogs significantly influences the microbial communities on the human hand that touches them regularly [33, 34]. Research on animal owners in Madagascar in Africa found out the connection between human skin and animal skin microbes. As expected, the animal skin microbiota was established to be more similar to its owner's body parts [35]. Animal owner and non-owner body parts after comparison were found to be made up of similar proportions of *Proteobacteria*, *Actinobacteria, Bacteroidetes, Firmicutes* (the four dominant human skin bacterial phyla) and *Cyanobacteria* [36]. In contrast, their animals were majorly dominated by *Proteobacteria* (88.5%). Animal owner's skins were found to have higher proportions of *Actinobacteria* and *Firmicutes*. The authors further found out that contact with the animal might not really be a major driver of skin microbial communities on their owners. This is because, certain bacterial taxa may be better suited to colonising human skin than animal skin, perhaps based on differences attributed to factors such as hair, sweat glands, pH or host genetics [37]. These findings suggest that interactions within the shared environment of all humans, regardless of animal ownership, can homogenise the skin microbiome, but that different body sites may harbour distinct microbial communities due to dispersal from environmental microbes [37, 38].

Animal hides and skins could also act as a mechanism for the transmission of bacteria and other microbes, due to its high content of moisture and nutrients (carbohydrates, fats, and proteins). These raw materials for making leather also contribute to the indoor environment of a tannery. The indoor environment inside the tanning industry has been associated with some human diseases attributed to biological agents. Conducted studies report that livestock and tannery workers have contracted diseases such as *Tetanus, Anthrax, Leptospirosis, 'Q' fever, Brucellosis, afta epizootic, Dermatosis and Micotoxicosis* due to infection and contamination of raw hide or skin, poor working conditions and to some extent processed leather. In addition, the above, genuses of fungi have also been reported in this environment, and they include species such as *Aspergillus niger* and *Penicillium glaucum*. Yeast genera that include *Rhodotorula, Cladosporium Torulopsis* have also been reported. Prolonged exposure of tannery workers to the tannery environment and their processed products has been closely linked with the development of allergies and asthma as well as the long-term exposure to fungi microbes. This ends up in the development of respiratory infections and other diseases [39]. For example, in Bangladesh, the common health problems diagnosed among the tannery workers were reported as shown in **Table 1**.

On the other hand, it would be interesting to determine if the above-mentioned taxa, are transient members of the human skin community as a result of temporary contact between the human body and this animal by-product, or it is due to long-term contact with animals and their products (and the shared environment) results in fundamental shifts in human skin communities that allow taxa that are typically considered animal and their products microbes to become residents [41]. When a beneficial microbe of animal skin is transferred to the human skin through the use of leather products, where there are a resident species of the same genera, what happens between the introduced species and indigenous microbes is still unknown. For example, *Bacillus subtilis* is known to protect the skin against other microbes.

Diseases reported among tannery workers	Number of cases reported (%)
Asthma	138 (49.9)
Diarrhoea	198 (71.7)
Jaundice/typhoid	120 (43.5)
Blood pressure	144 (52.2)
Gastrointestinal problem	198 (71.7)
Eye problem	129 (46.7)
Scabies	204 (73.9)
Nail discoloration	192 (69.6)
Urticaria	165 (59.7)
Miliaria and folliculitis	156 (56.6)
Contact dermatitis	108 (39.13)
Sores	105 (38.04)
Pruritus	90 (32.61)
Hand eczema	81 (29.35)
Fungal infection	75 (27.2)

Table 1.
Prevalence of diseases including occupational dermatitis among tannery workers of Bangladesh (adapted from Mahamudul [40]).

What happens when the one from animal skin/leather product is introduced into the human skin which is occupied by resident human *Bacillus subtilis*?. This is still unclear and provides an area worth looking into in future studies of the leather microbiome. This is because it is not known whether they live mutually, commensally, compete or they kill one another to get or retain the space. Clear explanation about this interaction is now necessary considering the fact that leather plays a basic role in human daily life.

5. Possible reported ways to hinder the transmission pathway of microbes to humans

The microorganisms grow on raw hides firstly because of their ability to hydrolyse the proteins present. This is due to their proteolysis degrading effect of the raw hide/skin substance [42]. In the literature, various authors have shown concern with halophilic micro-organisms and the problem of the colouration of cured hides/skins. The role of halophilic and non-halophilic bacteria producing or not producing coloured spots on salted hide/skin is still not yet clear, because the individual types can manifest themselves successively to a point that their individual hydrolytic effects are hidden from detection by various methods. Various bacterial species isolated from fresh calf skins are reported to have the ability to withstand a high level of salt (NaCI) concentrations (1.5–9% w/v) [42]. These isolated bacterial species included *Bacillus coli*, *Bacillus proteus*, *Bacillus megaterium*, *Bacillus mycoides*, *Bacillus subtilis*, *Staphylococcus albus*, *Staphylococcus aureus*, *Sarcina lutea* and *Micrococcus roseus*. *Bacillus subtilis* and *Bacillus mycoides* were found to survive in the dormant state at a high salt concentration (20% w/v) [42]. Bacteria called *Mesophiles*, such as *tuberculosis* known to be causing *Mycobacterium tuberculosis* can survive best at normal room temperature and are likely to thrive longer than cold-loving *Psychrophiles* or heat-loving *Thermophiles*. Other microbes do form exoskeleton-like spores as a defence mechanism, like the bacteria called *Staphylococcus aureus*. It is responsible for toxic shock syndrome and wound infections. The *Bacillus anthracis*, anthrax-causing bacteria, can also form spores and survive tens to hundreds of years [6]. The use of salt as a bacteriostat is to inhibit the growth of these microbes on the green hides and skin in curing premises.

When converting skin into finished leather, collagen which is the basic fibre component must be protected since many characteristics of finished leather, particularly its durability, rely on collagen protein. Thus, bactericides with a broad spectrum are widely preferred in the main soaking process to stop bacterial attacks. However, fungi and bacteria displaying proteolytic and lipolytic activities at a remarkable level on raw hides and skins and in the pre-tanning floats should be taken into consideration and monitored. This is due to, the fact that these microbes are able to survive in extreme conditions [43]. A number of bacterial species such as *Bacillus sp.*, *Pseudomonas sp.*, *Alcaligenes sp.*, *Escherichia coli*, and *Shewanella alga* are reported to have Cr^{6+} detoxification capability due to the presence of reductases enzyme soluble in cytosol [44]. In *Pseudomonas maltophilia* and *Bacillus megaterium*, the Cr^{6+} reduction is associated with membrane cell fractions [16]. However, at present, it is still unclear whether the reduction of Cr^{5+} to Cr^{4+} and Cr^{4+} to Cr^{3+} is coordinated or enzymes regulated process. The NADH, NADPH, and electrons from the endogenous reservoir are suspected to be the electron donors in the Cr^{6+} reduction process. However, unlike Cr^{6+} reductases enzymes isolated from aerobes microbes, the Cr^{6+} reducing activities of anaerobes microbes are associated with their electron transfer systems ubiquitously catalysing the electron shuttle alone [16]. During the reduction reaction, the enzyme Cr^{6+} reductase (ChrR) transiently reduces Cr^{6+} with a one-electron shuttle reaction to form Cr^{5+} followed by a two-electron transfer to form Cr^{3+} [46]. Although a proportion of the Cr^{5+} intermediate is spontaneously reoxidised to generate reactive oxygen species (ROS), its reduction reaction through two-electron transfer catalysed by ChrR reduces the chances to produce harmful radicals which can harm the cell. Several facultative anaerobes such as *Pseudomonas dechromaticans, Pseudomonas chromatophila, Aeromonas chromatica, Mycobacterium spp, Geobacter metallireducens, Shewanella putrefaciens, Pantoea agglomerans*, and *Agrobacterium radiobacter* EPS-916 are also reported to catalyse the biotransformation change of Cr^{6+} to Cr^{3+} under anoxic conditions [45].

Biodeterioration is reported to be an important factor that can impair aesthetic, functional and other properties of leather and other biopolymers or organic materials and the products made from them globally. This process takes place particularly under conditions of high relative humidity that enable bacteria, actinomycetes fungi or other microbes to grow fast [15]. Biodeterioration in the leather industry has been mentioned to results from the activity of macro- and micro-organisms on raw hides and skins, during leather manufacture and also during storage of finished leathers and leather articles [20, 46, 47]. Because of its protein and lipids nature, leather provides a suitable substrate for many micro-organisms. The biodeterioration process also happens on detanning (removal of chrome tannin on leather) effect and growth of *Penicillium spp*. The cross-link between collagen protein and chromium tanning agent is weakened during the biodeterioration reaction. It is speculated that protease enzymes that are produced by the *Penicillium spp* could be the degrading agent for chromium tanned leather. At the beginning of biodeterioration reaction, the *Penicillium spp* could be using the uncross-linked collagen protein as nourishment to grow and multiply, leading to the damaging of the collagen molecule. The *Penicillium spp* growth and multiplication makes tanning effect much weaker and susceptible. The detanned chromium leather becomes much easier for the *Penicillium spp* digesting enzymes and the biodeterioration begin slowly until the whole leather is affected completely [48].

In most cases, the *Pseudomonas spp* are normally present on the skin surface. Fur and skin layer might also contribute to the *Bacillus spp*. The presence of antibiotic-resistant plasmid harbouring *E.coli* has also been reported in leather and leather products [49]. *Staphylococcus aureus* generally has been present in epidermal and dermal layers of the animal's skin. These isolates were detected to have antigenic structures that enable them to resist antibiotics. The resistance development may be due to the nonspecific mechanism with gene regulation of plasmids and chromosomes, which may be heritable or transferable due to the presence of the resistance factor (R-factor) [49]. These structures enable the microbes to withstand extreme alkalinity and acidity in the tanning process; as such these microbes pose a real health hazard to the tannery workers.

Various studies have been carried out in order to develop clean or cleaner technologies to reduce the pollution load during leather manufacturing processes. These clean and cleaner technologies are also known by other name as best available technologies (BAT) [50]. Initially, it was assumed that the replacement of hazardous chemicals with non-hazardous chemicals may provide suitable conditions for microbial growth because of the shift in pH concentration. The growth and survival of micro-organisms, particularly pathogenic bacteria related to health issues, at various stages of the leather manufacturing processes (both conventional and BAT) has been investigated using *Bacillus cereus, Pseudomonas aeruginosa,* and *Staphylococcus*. At the end of the study, no considerable differences were observed between the effect of the conventional and BAT leather making processes on these bacterial growths. This study confirmed one fundamental issue of interest and concern, that is, the ability of bacterial cells to recover and regenerate during leather manufacture [50]. This is an important point to note when dealing with processed leather and leather products and their relation to the health of tannery workers.

Careful consideration is still necessary regarding pathogen-related health issues even though the bacterial (*Bacillus cereus, Pseudomonas aeruginosa*, and *Staphylococcus*) counts were found to be low in processed leather. This is because, the risk of bacterial infections in humans may depend on many other factors, such as the tannery environment, the leather making procedures and the personnel involved in leather making processes. There is a likelihood that pathogenic bacteria may still be present and caution is recommended when dealing with hides/skins and leather products at any stage. Growth and proliferation of fungi in the hide/skin and leather products also still require investigation, as various studies have shown that leather production may provide suitable conditions for fungal growth as BAT studies reported here did not include fungal study [51]. In addition to the above mentioned, areas for further qualitative and quantitative analysis is required to determine the presence of microorganisms in the tannery based solid waste as well, such as sludge, the fleshing, shavings, hair, buffing dust, and trimmings which are generated during leather processing. This is due to the fact that these wastes are now being recycled into different products and used for different purposes by the general populace.

6. Pathogenic microbes on humans and on the leather products

Although the majority of the isolated microbial species are non-harmful and do not cause infections to humans, studies also show that some species in the genera *Bacillus, Staphylococcus, Pseudomonas, Klebsiella, Aspergillus,* and *Candida* are considered pathogens or potential pathogens [52]. These microbes and others associated with animal skin and leather product cause diseases in human. For example, *Escherichia coli* and *Enterobacter species* can cause urinary tract infection, wound infection and abscesses septicaemia. *Lactobacilli species* are a rare cause of septicaemia, endocarditis, and meningitis [52]. *Staphylococcus epidermidis, Staphylococcus aureus* is the most common microbes found on the human skin and nose. About 25% of healthy people in the world carry these bacteria, according to the Centre for Disease Control and Prevention (CDC). *Staphylococcus* bacteria coexist peacefully on our body. If a person with low immunity gets the infection from someone else's *Staphylococcus*, the bacteria can cause nasty skin infections, and pneumonia [52].

Klebsiella species may cause urinary tract infection, respiratory infection, and septicaemia. *Klebsiella pneumoniae, Klebsiella oxytoca, Klebsiella granulomatis* bacteria are generally found in human intestines, where they generally exist peacefully with others. However, different types of the bacteria can spread in the body and cause infection in sick patients in hospital environment, including pneumonia, blood infections, skin infections, and meningitis. *Haemophilus influenza* bacteria was mistakenly believed to be the culprit behind flu virus outbreaks long ago when it was first discovered in 1892. While most strains do not cause disease in humans, the bacteria can cause respiratory tract and heart valve infections and sexually transmitted chancre sores in those with weakened immune systems [52, 49]. *Streptococcus mitis, Streptococcus salivarius, Streptococcus mutans, Streptococcus pneumonia, Streptococcus pyogenes* bacteria range greatly in their potential to cause disease and how they are spread in the environment. Group A of the *Streptococcus*, generally lives harmoniously in the throat or on the skin but can cause mild illnesses such as strep throat and skin infections. Group B of *Streptococcus* infections tend to be more severe and are more common in older or sick adults with the weak immune system. Group B infections are reported to be the leading cause of meningitis and blood infections in newborn children.

Neisseria gonorrhoeae, Neisseria meningitidis, Neisseria lactamica, Neisseria cinerea, Neisseria polysaccharea, Neisseria mucosa, Neisseria flavescens, Neisseria sicca, Neisseria subflava, Neisseria elongata, Neisseria gonorrhoeae and *Neisseria meningitidis* are bacteria that live in humans. Only two *Neisseria spp* causes disease. These types are most notoriously known for causing meningitis and gonorrhoeae, which thrive in mucous membranes and they are normally spread through sexual contact. *Neisseria* generally live in the upper respiratory tract and are not harmful to humans. *Bacteroides caccae, Bacteroides distasonis, Bacteroides eggerthii, Bacteroides fragilis, Bacteroides merdae, Bacteroides ovatus, Bacteroides stercoris, Bacteroides thetaiotaomicron, Bacteroides uniformis, Bacteroides vulgatus* bacteria have a complicated relationship with humans [52, 49]. When they are isolated from the gut, they assist in breaking down food and synthesising nutrients and energy for the body to use. When they escape the intestines, they can cause deadly infections in the blood and even form abscesses all over the body which is normally seen on the skin as signs of infection.

Clostridium perfringens, Clostridium difficile, Clostridium tetani (only transiently associated with humans, do not colonise the intestines) bacteria are commonly found in the soil and human intestines, and generally do not cause problems. A few strains of *clostridium* can produce potent toxins, including botulism, tetanus, and an irritation of the intestines and cause a mild to a life-threatening illness called *Clostridium difficile*, which causes inflammation of the intestines. *Mycobacterium* bacteria is most notorious for causing severe illnesses such as tuberculosis, leprosy, and Hansen's disease, though most species of *Mycobacteria* in nature are benign in humans, unless in cases of those who have weakened immune systems. The *Pseudomonas aeruginosa* microbe is extremely versatile and can live in a wide range of environments, including soil, water, animals, plants, sewage, and hospitals in addition to humans. It seldom makes healthy people sick, but more typically causes blood infections and pneumonia in those who are hospitalised or have weakened immune systems. *Mycoplasmas* are particularly tricky to detect, diagnose, and eradicate in the human body. Though *Mycobacteria* belong to the normal flora in humans, most species of *Mycobacteria* are harmful and can cause respiratory and urinary tract infections [52, 49]. Thus microbes found in animal skins and are able to survive through the leather tanning process and reach human skin might cause diseases in people with weak immune system.

7. Conclusion

The most common bacteria found growing on leather purses are *Micrococcus* and *Staphylococcus* species each accounting for around two-thirds, followed by *Bacillus* (14%). *Micrococcus* was found to be more common on the men's purses, while *Bacillus* was found only on women's purses. In general, the study found out that the most common bacteria and fungus prevalence in leather are *Micrococcus, Bacillus, Staphylococcus, Aspergillus spp, Trichoderma* and *Penicillium spp*. Some are non-harmful and do not cause infections in humans. Other species within the genera of *Bacillus, Staphylococcus, Pseudomonas, Klebsiella, Aspergillus,* and *Candida* are pathogens or potential pathogens; therefore, they need to be monitored and controlled in skin and leather products to avoid their cross transfer as they can spread diseases in human. Thus, further studies on "leather microbiome" are of the essence to human health and disease.

The Role of Leather Microbes in Human Health
DOI: http://dx.doi.org/10.5772/intechopen.81125

Acknowledgements

I acknowledge God for giving me strength to write this piece of work and the support of my promoters.

Conflict of interest

I don't have any conflict of interest in this work.

Author details

Richard O. Oruko*, John O. Odiyo and Joshua N. Edokpayi
Department of Hydrology and Water Resources, University of Venda,
Thohoyandou, South Africa

*Address all correspondence to: richardoruko@gmail.com

IntechOpen

References

[1] American Museum of Natural History Human Microbiome. The Role of Microbes in Human Health. 2016. https://www.readworks.org/article/ Human-Microbiome-The-Role-of-Microbes-in-Human-Health/d558946f-2097-4d58-8008-e19e00beb355#!articleTab:content/

[2] Kumar A, Chordia N. Role of microbes in human health. Application Microbiology Open Access. 2017;**3**:2. DOI: 10.4172/2471-9315.1000131

[3] Cogen AL, Nizet V, Gallo RL. Skin microbiota: A source of disease or defence. The British Journal of Dermatology. 2008;**158**:442-455

[4] Johnson TJ. The Animal Microbiome in Health and Disease. University of Minnesota Twin Cities St. Paul, United States: Frontiers Media S.A. All Rights Reserved. 2008. https://www. frontiersin.org/research-topics/6881/ the-animal-microbiome-in-health-and-disease

[5] Battelli G. Zoonoses as occupational diseases. Veterinaria Italiana. 2008;**44**(4):601-609

[6] Melik J, Ethirajan A. Anthrax outbreak hits Bangladesh leather and meat sectors. Reporters, Business Daily, BBC World Service. 2010. https://www. bbc.com/news/business-11451570

[7] Centre for Disease Prevention. Exposure to Hides/Drums. 2015. https:// www.cdc.gov/anthrax/specificgroups/ animal-workers/hides-drums.html

[8] Bielak E, Cholewińska JS. Antimicrobial effect of lining leather fatliquored with the addition of essential oils. Biotechnology and Food Science. 2017;**4**:30-33

[9] Ruhrmann U. Microbiological studies on the occurrence of micrococcaceae in slaughter cattle. The Veterinary Record. 1987;**178**:17

[10] Mohamed HAA, Van Klink EGM, El Hassan SM. Damage caused by spoilage bacteria to the structure of cattle hides and sheep skins. International Journal of Animal Health and Livestock Production Research. 2016;**2**(1):39-56

[11] Holt JC, Krieg NR, Sneath PHA, Stalley JT, Williams ST. Bergey's Manual of Determinative Bacteriology. 9th ed. Philadelphia: Lippincott Williams and Wilkins; 1994

[12] Barrow GL, Feltham RKA. Cowan and Steel's Manual for Identification of Medical Bacteria. 3rd ed. Cambridge, UK: Cambridge University Press; 1993

[13] Kayalvizhi N, Anthony T, Gunasekaran P. Characterization of predominant bacteria in cattle hides and their control by a bacteriocin. Journal of the American Leather Chemists Association. 2008;**103**(6):182-187

[14] Orlita A. Microbial biodeterioration of leather and its control: A review. International Biodeterioration & Biodegradation. 2004;**53**:157-163

[15] Bitlisli BO, Karavana HA, Baaran B, Sarı Ö, Birbir M. The effect of conservation defects on the suede quality of doubleface. Journal of the American Leather Chemists Association. 2004;**99**:494-501

[16] Nigam RK. Environmental mycology of tannery unit (TEFCO-lime section) at Kanpur—Allergical aspects. In: 5th Aerobiology-International Conference, 1994, Bangalore. https://docplayer. net/55453841-Microorganisms-isolated-and-antimicrobial-treatments-applied-at-different-stages-of-leather-processing.html

[17] Ozdilli K, Işsever H, Ozyildirim BA, Hapeloqlu B, Ince N, Ince H, et al.

Biological hazards in tannery workers. Indoor and Built Environment. 2007;**16**(4):349-357

[18] Srinath T, Verma T, Ramteke PW, Garg SK. Chromium (VI) biosorption and bioaccumulation by chromate resistant bacteria. Chemosphere. 2002;**48**:427-435

[19] Wang RR, Li CX, Xu BB, Liang L, Li YH, Peng BY. Isolation of moulds from wet-blue leathers and the investigation of the influence of environmental conditions on the growth of typical moulds. Leather Science and Engineering. 2012;**22**:5e11

[20] Ozgunay H, Cadircia BH, Vurala C, yilmazb O. A new defect on leather: microbial bio-film. American Leather Chemists. 2010. https://www.researchgate.net/ publication/221787877_A_New_Defect_ On_Leather_Microbial_BioFilm

[21] Orlita A. Microbial biodeterioration of leather and its control. In: II Konferencja Naukowa: Rozkład i Korozja Mikrobiologiczna Materiałów Technicznych (in Polish). Łódź: Politechnika Łódzka; 2001. pp. 41-54

[22] Skóra J, Gutarowska B, Śnioszek A. Zanieczyszczenie mikrobiologiczne w garbarniach—zagrożenie dla przetwarzanego surowca, wyrobów skórzanych oraz zdrowia pracowników zakładów garbarskich. Vol. 1. Przegląd WOS; 2014. pp. 26-33. (in Polish). http:// yadda.icm.edu.pl/baztech/element/ bwmeta1.element.baztech-8068398d-8b88-4a43-b9d9-c23b9d20bde9

[23] Biranjia-Hurdoyal SD, Deerpaul S, Permal GK. A study to investigate the importance of purses as fomites. Advanced Biomedical Research. (published online). 2015. http://www. advbiores.net/article.asp?issn=2277-9175;year=2015;volume=4;issue=1; spage=102;epage=102;aulast=Biran jia-Hurdoyal

[24] Szostak-Kot J. Mikrobiologia produktów. Kraków: Wydawnictwo UEK; 2010. p. 122. (in Polish)

[25] Krzyściak P, Skóra M, Bulanda M. Epidemiologia grzybic paznokci na podstawie danych Zakładu Mykologii UJ-CM. In: Warsztaty Polskiego Towarzystwa Mykologicznego Grzyby—organizmy kluczowe dla życia na ziemi. Łódź-Spała; 2014. pp. 104-106. (in Polish). http://www.km.cm-uj.krakow.pl/ ogloszenia-dla-studentow/

[26] Glausiusz J. Your body is a planet, 90% of the cells within us are not ours but microbes. Discover Magazine. June issue. 2007. http://discovermagazine. com/2007/jun/your-body-is-a-planet

[27] Rosenberg Z, Rosenberg E. Role of microorganisms in the evolution of animals and plants: The hologenome theory of evolution. FEMS Microbiology Reviews. 2008;**32**(5):723-735. DOI: 10.1111/j.1574-6976.2008.00123.x

[28] Lori MC, Christopher RL, Stiles CM. Introduction to Fungi. Washington State University, Kansas State University, and Georgia Military College; 2012. Available from: https://www.researchgate. net/publication/230-0888186_ Introduction_to_Fungi [Accessed: Jun 20, 2018]. DOI: 10.1094/PHI-I-2012-0426-01. https://scholar. google.com/citations?user=CGbIx 50AAAAJ&hl=en#d=gs_md_cita-d&p=&u=%2Fcitations%3Fview_ op%3Dview_citation%26hl%3Den% 26user%3DCGbIx50AAAAJ%26citat ion_for_view%3DCGbIx50AAAAJ%3A efIP2zaiRacC%26 tzom%3D-120

[29] Song SJ, Lauber CL, Costello EK. Cohabiting family members share microbiota with one another and with their dogs. Microbiology and Infectious Disease. 2013;**eLIF**(2):e00458

[30] Melissa BM, Yu JJ, Lawrence PP, Olaf M, Sarah CW, Julie EH, et al. Environmental influences on the skin microbiome of humans and cattle in rural Madagascar. Evolution, Medicine, and Public Health. 2017;(1):144-153

[31] Caporaso JG, Flores GE, Henley JB. Temporal variability is a personalized feature of the human microbiome. Genome Biology. 2014;15:531

[32] Grice EA, Segre JA. The skin microbiome. Nature Reviews. Microbiology. 2011;9:244-253

[33] Grice EA, Kong HH, Conlan S. Topographical and temporal diversity of the human skin microbiome. Science. 2009;324:1190-1192

[34] Eberl L, Vandamme P. Members of the genus *Burkholderia*: Good and bad guys. F1000 Research. 2016;5(F1000 Faculty Rev):1007

[35] Hospodsky D, Pickering AJ, Julian TR. Hand bacterial communities vary across two different human populations. Microbiology. 2014;160:1144-1152

[36] Anderson H. The adaptation of various Bacteria to growth in the presence of sodium chloride. Journal of the Society of Leather Technologists and Chemists. 1945;24:215-217

[37] Reed A, Bergeron E. How long do microbes like bacteria and viruses live on surfaces in the home at normal room temperatures. 2002. https://www.popsci.com/scitech/article/2002-08/how-long-do-microbes-bacteria-and-viruses-live-surfaces-home-normal-room-tem

[38] Ali NY. The effect of using a fungicide along with bactericide in the main soaking float on microbial load. African Journal of Biotechnology. 2008;7(21):3922-3926

[39] Castellanos AP, Camarena-Pozos DA, Castellanos DC. Microbial contamination in the indoor environment of tanneries in Leon, Mexico. Indoor and Built Environment. 2015;25(3):1-17 (journals Permissions. nav). DOI: 10.1177/1420326X 14564798

[40] Mahamudul HMD, Hosain S, Asaduzzaman AM, Haque MA, Roy UK. Prevalence of health diseases among Bangladeshi tannery workers and associated risk factors with workplace investigation. Journal of Pollution Effects & Control. 2016;4:4. DOI: 10.4175/2375-4397. 1000175

[41] Bharagava RN, Yadav A, Mishra S, Kaithwas G, Raj A. Organic pollutants and pathogenic bacteria in tannery wastewater and their removal strategies. In: Microbes and Environmental Management. 2016. https://www.researchgate.net/profile/Ram_Naresh_Bharagava/publication/290709995_Organic_Pollutants_and_Pathogenic_Bacteria_in_Tannery_Wastewater_and_their_Removal_Strategies/links/56ee8e1b08ae4b8b5e74fbe9/Organic-Pollutants-and-Pathogenic-Bacteria-in-Tannery-Wastewater-and-their-Removal-Strategies.pdf

[42] Ackerley DF, Gonzalez CF, Keyhan M, Blake IIR, Matin A. Mechanism of chromate reduction by the *E. coli* protein, NfsA, and the role of different chromate reductases in minimizing oxidative stress during chromate reduction. Environmental Microbiology. 2004;6:851-860

[43] Orlita A. Biodeterioration of leather materials especially book-leather bindings and parchments. In: Garg KL, Garg N, Mukejri KG, editors. Recent Advances in Biodeterioration and Biodegradation. Vol. I. Calcutta, India: Naya Prokash; 1993. pp. 259-299

[44] Zyska B. Microbial Deterioration of Materials. Warszawa, Poland: WN-T; 1997. pp. 181-200

[45] Zhang J, Zhangwei H, Teng B, Chen W. Biodeterioration process of chromium tanned leather with Penicillium sp. International Biodeterioration & Biodegradation. 2017. https://www.infona.pl/resource/bwmeta1.element.elsevier-bd7f8ff3-889b-3937-a496-765cbe7fa888

[46] Shanthi J, Saravanan T, Balagurunathan R. Isolates of tannery effluent and their antibiogram from effluent plant. South India Journal of Chemical and Pharmaceutical Research. 2012;4(4):1974-1977

[47] Lama A. The impact of the leather manufacturing process on bacterial growth [doctoral thesis]. The University of Northampton; 2010

[48] Wilson J. Clinical Microbiology, an Introduction for Healthcare Professionals. Edinburgh: Bailliere Tindall; 2005

[49] Kerr JR. Bacterial inhibition of fungal growth and pathogenicity. Microbial Ecology in Health and Disease. 1999;11(3):129-142. DOI: 10.1080/089106099435709

[50] Hanlin MB, Field RA, Ray B, Bailey DG. Characterization of predominant bacteria in cattle hides and their control by a Bacteriocin. Journal of the American Leather Chemists Association. 1995;90(10):282-321

[51] Higgins MJ, Chen Y-C, Murthy SN, Hendrickson D, Farrel J, Schafer P. Reactivation and growth of non-culturable indicator bacteria in anaerobically digested biosolids after centrifuge dewatering. Water Research. 2007;41(3):665-673

[52] Calderone J. 13 creepy pictures of the microbes that are living inside of you. 2015. https://www.businessinsider.com.au/microbiome-human-bacteria-gut-intestine-mouth-skin-2015-11#/#genus-staphylococcus-1

Chapter 4

Extra Pulmonary Tuberculosis: An Overview

Onix J. Cantres-Fonseca, William Rodriguez-Cintrón,
Francisco Del Olmo-Arroyo and Stella Baez-Corujo

Abstract

Mycobacterium tuberculosis is the bacterium that as a single agent is known to cause the infection with the most morbidity and mortality around the world. It is known to cause pulmonary infection in immunocompetent patient, but its dissemination outside the lungs has been linked to a high degree of cellular immunosuppression as seen in the advance stages of human immunodeficiency virus infection, and after chemotherapy. Despite extensive research, screening, education, and continuous efforts to try to eradicate and control the infection, tuberculosis is still one of the most prevalent infections throughout the world. Even the cases of extra pulmonary dissemination are seen to have increased. Extra pulmonary tuberculous dissemination has a very variable presentation that depends on the organ involved. The diagnosis is difficult and many times a long time passes between diagnosis and initial presentation. In this chapter, we will review how tuberculosis infection presents when the bacilli invades any tissue outside the pulmonary parenchyma, what the literature recommends for the proper work up and diagnosis, and general treatment for major organ system infection.

Keywords: tuberculosis, extra pulmonary, infection, mycobacterium

1. Introduction

Although it is well known that *Mycobacterium tuberculosis* can be pathologic to any organ system, its manifestations can be so variable that sometimes it becomes a challenge for the clinician to identify or even consider it as the cause of the patient's symptomatology. Most of the times, an extensive work up with invasive interventions is required for proper diagnosis.

Extra pulmonary tuberculosis (EPTB), described this way when the tuberculous mycobacterium invades areas outside the pulmonary parenchyma, has nonspecific clinical findings developing insidiously [1] mimicking other noninfectious conditions [2]. It requires a high clinical suspicion and carries a lengthy period from the initial symptoms to the final diagnosis.

Nevertheless, its presentation can be extremely acute causing a life threatening condition [1]. Clinical presentation will vary according to the organ system involved and more than one organ could be involved at the same time. The initial step in early identification is having knowledge of its findings in the proper clinical setting and including them within the differential diagnosis. Even though some patients do not have the expected risk factors, tuberculosis is identified as the culprit of symptoms associated with other conditions.

This illustrates the ample spectrum of extra-pulmonary tuberculosis manifestations. Vast medical knowledge helps the clinician to identify this condition in the adequate clinical scenario to pursue its diagnosis.

In this chapter, a review of the most important clinical manifestations of extra-pulmonary tuberculosis will be discussed. It will also review the required work up and specific treatment for other organs involved.

2. Epidemiology

Mycobacterium tuberculosis, as a single infectious agent, causes more deaths than any other infection [3]. Outside infectious diseases, it is the ninth leading cause of death worldwide [3]. According to the World Health Organization (WHO) and the Global Tuberculosis report, in 2016, the largest incidence of tuberculosis occurred in areas of Korea and Africa [3]. In 2016, more than 10 millions of people were infected with tuberculosis around the world [3]. Active tuberculosis occurs in approximately 10% of the infected patients, involving lung parenchyma only in approximately 85% of subjects [7], but the incidence of other organ involvement varies widely in endemic and nonendemic areas.

Worldwide, the incidence of extra-pulmonary involvement of tuberculosis occurs in approximately 17–52% of all cases reported [4]. In other publications, the incidence from reported cases varies from 15 to 40%, with approximately 3–3.5 cases per 100,000 of the population from 2002 to 2011 [5]. Although, the incidence has been stable or decreased in some areas, a report from 2003 to 2008 showed an increased worldwide incidence from 30.6 to 37.6% secondary to longer life expectancy of immunosuppressed patients due to better medical care [6]. In the United States, the incidence of EPTB increased from 15.7% of the cases in 1993 to 21.0% in 2006 [8]. Therefore, EPTB continues to be an important presentation within tuberculosis infectious spectrum.

The demography of EPTB cases varies widely among documented case series. A review published in *Clinical Infectious Diseases* in 2009 [6] revealed that from 253,299 of tuberculosis cases reported in the USA from 1999 to 2006, 19% were extra pulmonary, while 8% were disseminated or concurrently pulmonary and EPTB. The mean age of this group was 44 years old, with a proportion of male to female almost one to one. Children (described in this population as less than 15 years old) with reported EPTB were approximately 6% of the cases. This same publication revealed predominance of genitourinary and bone and joint involvement in older patients (more than 60-year old), while children accounted for most of the cases of meningeal and lymphatic involvement.

3. Organ involvement

Tuberculosis can invade practically any organ. The proportions of organ involved in multiple publications suggest that most extra pulmonary tuberculous cases are seen with pleural, bone, and lymphatic involvement [6, 9]. In rare cases, the involvement can be localized to a specific organ [2], while 2–10% of the cases are reported to be disseminated within more than two organ systems [6, 9]. Most cases occur secondary to activation of previous pulmonary contagion.

4. Risk factors

Multiple populations with tuberculosis have been studied. In a case series described by García-Rodríguez et al., the mean age of patients with EPTB was higher than patients with pulmonary disease [6]. EPTB cases increased with the age, but the anatomical sites varied according to the age [6]. More cases of lymphatic, joint, and bone involvement were seen as patients become older. The female to male ratio varied according to the organ involvement, but in general, the male to female ratio was similar to other publications, which was one to one.

Although immunosuppression seen to be a risk factor for EPTB, a study published in *International Journal Tuberculosis Lung Disease* in 2009 suggested that diabetes mellitus was a risk factor for pulmonary tuberculosis, but not for EXPTB [10]. The protective mechanism for extra pulmonary dissemination of tuberculosis is known. The same study concluded that patients with end stage renal disease had a predisposition for EPTB. A possible mechanism that increases the risk for dissemination is a decrease cell-mediated immune response.

Other risk factors identified for extra-pulmonary dissemination include cirrhosis, malignancy, immunosuppressive drug use, alcoholism, HIV infection, chronic obstructive pulmonary disease (COPD), congestive heart failure, intravenous drug use, previous history of pulmonary tuberculosis, and history of cerebrovascular accident. There is not statistical analysis that linked all those causes as a direct risk factor for disseminated infection [10].

Cell-mediated immunosuppression has been linked to the development of tuberculosis and an increased risk of dissemination. Multiple reports and publications have linked HIV infection to the risk of developing EPTB. Among HIV patients admitted due to tuberculosis, almost 50% have extra pulmonary involvement [11]. Concomitant pulmonary and multi-organ involvement is common. Low counts of CD4 lymphocytic cells, which are in charge of cellular immune response, have been reported to be directly proportional to systemic dissemination, increasing the incidence of central nervous system (CNS) infection. Those patients with CNS involvement have higher mortality. Therefore, HIV infection predispose patients to EPT and its severity increase when CD4 levels decline to 200 cell/mm^3.

5. Pathophysiology

Tuberculosis infection is caused by aerobic bacteria, *Mycobacterium tuberculosis*. Mycobacteria have a cell wall with considerable amount of a fatty acid, mycolic acid, attached to a peptidoglycan-bound polysaccharide arabinogalactan, which provide a strong barrier resistant to antibiotics and (natural) defense mechanisms [12]. Pulmonary tuberculosis is acquired throughout airborne droplets that get into lungs and lead to pulmonary infection. Most of the bacteria are trapped in alveolar macrophages and destroyed. The mechanism of macrophages engulfment includes complement cascade activation when protein C3 binds to the cell wall and enhances recognition of the mycobacteria by macrophages. Mycobacterium phagocytosis initiates a cascade of events that results in either successful control of the infection, followed by latent tuberculosis, or progression to active disease.

After macrophage engulfment, they present the mycobacteria to T cell lymphocytes, which generate the formation of granulomas around the organisms. Granulomas have low levels of nutrients that restrict mycobacteria growth and therefore control the infection. Those patients with decreased immune response fail to control the infection and develop primary pulmonary infection. In patients infected, droplets produced during coughing can further spread the infection to other patients. Dissemination of the mycobacteria to other organ systems can occur when the bacilli get into a blood vessel or throughout the lymphatic system.

Reports suggest that most tuberculous empyemas and patients with vertebral bone involvement (Pott's disease) develop after the transport of tubercle bacilli from the pleural spaces to the parasternal and the para-aortic lymph nodes and the breakdown of caseous foci in these nodes [13]. These reports also explain investigations in which guinea pigs were injected with various doses of virulent tubercle bacilli inside their pleural cavity, developing granulomas in the liver, parasternal and para-aortic lymph nodes, spleen and kidneys, suggesting systemic dissemination. It all begins after the pleural space is invaded, disseminating to the thoracic lymph nodes and blood vessels, further seeding in distant organs.

6. Tuberculosis and organ system involvement

6.1 Central nervous system

Central nervous system tuberculous involvement occurs in approximately 5–10% of extra pulmonary cases [14]. It is a rare disease within the whole tuberculosis spectrum. This presentation has the most dangerous and catastrophic consequences.

Developing of CNS tuberculous infection has been linked to decreased cellular immune response as seen in HIV patients, malnutrition, alcoholism, malignancies, and the use of immunosuppressive agents [14]. Children and adolescents are more commonly involved with meningitis as the clinical presentation compared to adults (>15-year-old patients). In a study published in 2011, the mean age of patients with meningeal involvement is reported to be lower than those patients with infection in other organs such as lymphatic, bone and/or joint, and genitourinary [6].

Cases of EPTB are more common in older patients; however, a study from 2011 suggested that patients with ages less than 15 years old accounted for 5.4% of all TB patients. Although children were less likely to have EPTB, 13.8% of them presented as meningitis [6]. Peak of meningeal presentation was higher in patients younger than 24-year old. However, another study suggests that 40–70% of children with meningeal tuberculous involvement were exposed by older patients [15]. Risk factors related to meningitis by tuberculosis in children are similar to those related to infections in other sites, most cases related to some kind of immunosuppression. Median age of young patients with meningitis is approximately 4 y/o, and it is uncommon for children less than 6 months old to present with meningitis [15].

The most common clinical presentation of central nervous system involvement is meningitis. Most patients present with a history of nonspecific symptoms as malaise, anorexia, fatigue, fever, myalgia, and headache for approximately 2–8 weeks prior to the development of meningeal irritation [14]. In addition, neck rigidity and typical meningitis symptoms are more common in adults. These symptoms include depressed consciousness and nonspecific behavioral changes [14]. Tuberculosis can also cause focal nervous system deficits. Intracranial tuberculoma is the least common presentation. They are mass-like lesions that can be found in 1% of extra pulmonary patients with cerebral involvement and present with symptoms and signs of focal neurological deficit without the evidence of systemic disease [17]. Involvement of the spine occurs in less than 1% of TB patients, and it can be secondary to subjacent bone or soft tissue involvement [14]. Approximately 10% of patients with CNS tuberculosis have evidence of pulmonary tuberculosis [16].

Diagnosis of intracranial mycobacterium tuberculosis infection requires cerebral spinal fluid (CSF) cultures or acid fast stains obtained by spinal tap or tissue biopsy. Rates of CSF culture positivity for clinically diagnosed cases range from 25 to 70% [14]. In some cases, large volume spinal tap is required for diagnosis. However, HIV patients usually require less amount of fluid for diagnosis. Drug sensitivity testing is important for appropriate treatment. CSF sensitivity for culture and smear staining decrease significantly after treatment has been started [14], for which rapid diagnosis is essential to warrant the best outcome.

Polymerase chain reaction for *Mycobacterium tuberculosis* has also been used with variable results. Moreover, tuberculin skin tests and interferon gamma release assays could suggest exposure, but has limited utility for active disease diagnosis. Cerebral spinal fluid analysis for adenosine deaminase protein (ADA), an enzyme produced by lymphocytic proliferation differentiation during cell-mediated immunity, has also variable sensitivity for CNS infection. But standardized cutoffs have not been established. It has been used to predict CNS infection sequel that suggests poor outcomes in patients with higher values [14]. However, ADA levels in CNS can be high in other infections and noninfectious CNS pathologies. Therefore, correct diagnosis still requires CSF or tissue sample for AFB stains and cultures for mycobacterium.

Prompt therapy initiation with intravenous medications is extremely important for the treatment of tuberculous meningitis. First, line therapy for tuberculous CNS infection includes a combination of isoniazid, rifampicin, pyrazinamide, and ethambutol, which has to be taken daily. The recommended minimum duration is 10 months of therapy, which can be extended to 12 months if any interruption occurs during therapy. All medications have good hematoencephalic penetrance. On the other hand, monotherapy is not recommended due to the risk of developing an antimycobacterial therapy resistance, especially with isoniazid.

CNS lesions causing mass effect and hydrocephalus may require neurosurgical evaluation and cerebral decompression.

Systemic anti-inflammatory therapy with steroids should be started concomitantly (see **Table 1**). The use of anti-inflammatory medication has shown to decrease mortality without additional risk of adverse events [18]. Based on animal studies, the benefit of steroid therapy results from the reduction of the inflammatory process with a subsequent decrease in cerebral and spinal cord edema and brain pressure [18], with less disruptions in blood flow and cerebral perfusion.

In view of this, early diagnosis and initiation of antituberculous therapy with systemic steroids are vital to decrease mortality and improve outcome in patient with CNS tuberculous infection.

6.2 Thoracic extra pulmonary tuberculosis

It is believed that the development of extra pulmonary manifestation starts after mycobacterium bacilli invade pleural cavity from subjacent pulmonary parenchyma and then migrates to the lymphatic system, blood vessels, and eventually to other organs outside the thoracic cavity. For this reason is important to rule out pulmonary parenchymal tuberculosis when a patient is suspected to have a pleural effusion secondary to pleural invasion. Manifestations of tuberculosis in the pleural cavity could present either as pleural effusion or empyema. Pneumothorax as a result to parenchymal cavitary lesion rupture can also be seen. All pleural tuberculous involvements can end up in pleural tissue fibrosis or fibrothorax.

Fluid accumulates in the pleural cavity as a consequence of a hypersensitivity reaction to bacilli mycobacterium in the pleural space. Pleural tuberculosis occurs approximately in 5% of patient with tuberculosis in USA and can reach as high a 30% of patients within high prevalence populations [19]. Tuberculous pleural

Infection site	First line therapy	Duration	Adjunctive therapy
Central nervous system 1. Meningitis 2. Mass like lesion	1. Isoniazid, Rifampicin, Pyrazinamide* Isoniazid, Rifampicin, Pyrazinamide*	1. 9–12 months 2. 9–12 months	1. Systemic steroids 2. Surgical Resection (if mass effect or hydrocephalus)
Thoracic extra pulmonary tuberculosis 1. Tuberculous Pleurisy 2. Empyema	Isoniazid, Rifampicin, Pyrazinamide and Ethambutol	6 months	Percutaneous drainage or surgical evacuation
Gastrointestinal tuberculosis	Isoniazid, Rifampicin, Pyrazinamide and Ethambutol**	9–12 months	
Genitourinary tuberculosis	Isoniazid, Rifampicin, Pyrazinamide and Ethambutol	6–12 months (2 months of the 4 drugs followed by 4 months of Isoniazid and Rifampin)	Surgical resection in case of genito-urinary obstruction
Skeletal tuberculosis	Isoniazid, Rifampicin, Pyrazinamide and Ethambutol*	6–12 months (2 months of the 4 drugs followed by 4 months of Isoniazid and Rifampin)	Surgical resection in case of abscess formation or cord compression
Cutaneous tuberculosis	Isoniazid, Rifampicin, Pyrazinamide and Ethambutol	6–12 months	Colchicine, NSAID's, potassium iodine, dapsone, tetracyclines and antimalarial

Streptomycin can be added based in susceptibility.
**Therapy also can be based on susceptibility including Levofloxacin, Linezolid and Streptomycin.*

Table 1.
Extra pulmonary tuberculosis treatment.

effusions usually occur in the right side; these are small to moderate in size and are characterized as an exudate fluid. Fluid analysis is characterized with high protein levels (>5 g/dL), cell count around thousands, and lymphocytic predominance. It usually presents with more than 80% of lymphocytic predominance, and depending on the time of diagnosis, variable amounts of lymphocytes from 20 to 90% has been seen. In addition, low pH and low glucose levels can also be seen in pleural fluid analysis. Long standing effusions result in a highly acidic fluid. Lactate dehydrogenase enzyme (LDH) levels usually range above 500 IU/L [19].

Adenosine deaminase (ADA) levels (see CNS involvement) are of particular utility in suspected tuberculous pleural effusions. The diagnostic use of ADA depends on its sensitivity and specificity and the regional prevalence of the infection. In a high prevalence population, an elevated ADA level (>40 U/L) is considered confirmatory with a clear indication for therapy. In low prevalence populations, a low ADA level (<40 U/L) has a high negative predictive value and therefore, rules out the diagnosis [19]. There are cases where ADA levels are not considered reliable, for example, in patients with pulmonary, pleural or hematologic malignancies, nontuberculous bacterial infections and also in those who underwent pleural procedures.

Acid fast staining and culture test have limited diagnostic utility. Patients with pleural effusions of unknown etiology should be evaluated for a possible infectious cause, including tuberculosis. This is essential in patients with history of TB exposure, immunosuppression (including HIV), and pleural effusions with nonspecific characteristics, and lymphocytic cell count predominance.

Acid-fast smears are almost always negative. Positive cultures for mycobacterium tuberculosis have been reported in 10–70% of the cases [19], and consequently pleural fluid culture analysis has a low diagnostic yield. Positive culture is directly proportional to the level of immunosuppression. In an HIV patient, the yield doubles (20%) compared to the immunocompetent patient (10%). It is more common to obtain a positive culture in a liquid media versus solid media [19]. Positive pleural fluid cultures are useful for drug therapy sensitivity and should be obtained in every case of suspected tuberculous pleural effusion.

Pleural biopsy is considered one of the best diagnostic methods when tuberculous pleurisy is suspected. Definite diagnosis is obtained if mycobacterial bacillus is detected in the smear, culture or pleural tissue biopsy. In the appropriate clinical setting, the presence of granuloma obtained after pleural biopsy is highly suggestive of tuberculous pleurisy and demands treatment.

Percutaneous biopsy has a yield of almost 90% when guided by ultrasound [18]. When pleural biopsy is performed, the instruments and technique used varies, but the yield improves when at least six samples are taken from different quadrants [20]. More invasive procedures such as thoracoscopy and open surgical biopsies have good diagnostic yields. Access to these techniques is limited in areas of endemic tuberculosis, and for this reason, less invasive work up is the usual diagnostic approach. When a pleural effusion is suspected to be of tuberculosis origin, without evidence of pulmonary parenchymal involvement, a positive ADA in endemic areas is considered diagnostic. A low ADA level (<40) needs further work up including pleural biopsy. In low prevalence populations, a low ADA almost rules out tuberculosis and in these cases other etiologies must be considered [18].

Treatment for isolated pleural tuberculosis does not differ from pulmonary tuberculosis. Unless the effusion is characterized as an empyema, drainage is not required, and the effusion is expected to resolve by itself in weeks after commencement of treatment.

6.3 Gastrointestinal tuberculosis (abdominal tuberculosis)

Gastrointestinal tuberculosis (GI Tb) is relatively rare in the United States and is the sixth most common extrapulmonary location. Populations at risk include immigrants to the United States, the homeless, prisoners, residents of long-term care facilities, and the immunocompromised. The peritoneum and the ileocecal region are the most likely sites of infection and are involved in the majority of cases by hematogenous spread or through swallowing of infected sputum from primary pulmonary tuberculosis. Pulmonary tuberculosis is apparent in less than half of patients.

GI TB is a major health problem in many underdeveloped countries. In those with HIV infection, it is more present.

In those with pulmonary Tb, intestinal involvement was largely present before effective therapy was available.

However, approximately 20–25% of patients with GI TB have pulmonary TB. The ileum and colon are the common sites involved [21].

Other comorbidities associated with lower GI tract TB have been in other series type II diabetes mellitus (23%) and alcoholism (23%). Half of the stool cultures for *Mycobacterium tuberculosis* yields positive for it. This is similar to what is found with biopsy cultures of affected GI tract [22].

Treatment with 6 months antituberculous therapy has been found to be as effective as 9 months of therapy in patients with intestinal TB [23].

6.4 Specific situations

Esophageal Tb is the least common site of Tb in the GI tract [24]. *Stomach and duodenal* involvement by TB is rare because of (1) the high acidity of peptic secretions and (2) diminished amount of lymphoid tissue in the first part of the GI tract. Dyspepsia, diffuse abdominal pain, is frequent.

Clinical features of intestinal TB include abdominal pain, weight loss, anemia, and fever with night sweats. Patients may present with symptoms of obstruction, right sided pain [25].

Malabsorption may be caused by obstruction that leads to bacterial overgrowth, a variant of stagnant loop syndrome. Involvement of the mesenteric lymphatic system, known as tabes mesenterica, may retard chylomicron removal because of lymphatic obstruction and result in malabsorption.

The ileum is more commonly involved than the jejunum. Ileocecal involvement is seen in 80–90% of patients with GI TB. The latter is due to the abundance of lymphoid tissue in the distal ileum [26, 27].

If ascites is present, the measurement of ascitic fluid adenosine deaminase levels is reasonable. Laparoscopic biopsy samples from the peritoneum should be stained for acid-fast bacilli (AFB), and cultures should also be obtained with a reasonable yield [28, 29].

6.5 Genitourinary tuberculosis

Tuberculosis usually goes into the genitourinary system after reactivation of previous acquired disease. This is the second most common presentation of extra pulmonary disease, following lymphatic spread of infection [30]. Tuberculous bacilli infect renal and reproductive organs after they travel through the circulatory system. Genital involvement also occurs by cutaneous lesions during sexual contact or by contaminated instrumentation.

Genitourinary involvement mostly occurs after reactivation of latent disease, and time to reactivation occurs years after primary infection. Cases reported usually involve older patients with a median age above 40 year old and mostly affects male patients [23]. The urinary tract is usually involved and it can manifest as a simple cystitis or pyelonephritis with or without hematuria and renal failure.

When renal function is affected, the patient has urinary tract obstruction or an interstitial nephritis. The prostate, seminal vesicles, and epididymis are rarely affected. Epididymis is the most common genital organ involved in men followed by prostate [30]. Testicles involvement is very rare. In women, fallopian tubes and uterus are the most common genital organs involved and can cause infertility in small percent of young women [30].

Diagnosis is done showing evidence of bacilli in stain or cultures in urine or tissue obtained from the genitourinary tract. Granulomas and acid-fast bacilli can also be seen in tissue specimens from kidneys and reproductive organs [31]. Treatment is usually the same as pulmonary tuberculosis, with approximately 6–8 months as the recommended duration of therapy.

6.6 Skeletal tuberculosis

Skeletal tuberculosis presents with certain variability. It is responsible about 10% of all cases of extrapulmonary tuberculosis in the United States of America, with a highest prevalence among those immigrants who come from endemic areas. The proportion is no different between those patients infected with HIV versus those not infected. The most common affected area is the spine, follow tuberculous arthritis, and follow by extraspinal osteomyelitis. Young individuals are more likely to be affected in highly endemic are while adult patients are more frequently in low endemic together with a late presentation [32, 33].

The associated pathogenesis resides in disease confinement at the bone and the synovial fluid. It results after seeding during primary infection. Cellular and adaptive response are responsible of disease containment until reactivation which related to immunity failing which can be seen in different settings including older age, renal failure, malnutrition, and acquired immune deficiencies. Skeletal involvement shows histopathological pattern of caseous exudative or granular. The first occurs more frequently in children and it is characterized by inflammatory changes, bone destruction, abscess, and sinus tract formation. The last is much slower and much less destructive. Any bone can be infected with tuberculosis. Clinical manifestations include spondylitis, arthritis, and osteomyelitis [33, 34].

Tuberculous spondylitis (also known as Pott's disease) is the most common presentation. It is responsible for one half of the bone-related cases and most commonly affects the lower thorax and upper lumbar region. The infection starts at the anterior area of the vertebral joint and locally spreads to the anterior ligament after that it will affect the local vertebral body. Once the adjacent vertebra is affected, it proceeds to involve the intervertebral disk space with vertebral narrowing and further collapse. This finding may lead to distortion of the spinal canal anatomy and possible neurologic compromise. Although continuous spinal infection is uncommon, it has been documented [35]. Less than 40% of the patients presents with fever and weight loss. Symptoms include progressive local pain over the weeks with associated muscle spam and rigidity. The patient may present with an erect posture with associated short steps. Unfortunately, due to the lack of medical access on endemic regions, many of these patients will present with cord compression. Radiography changes are first appreciated in the anterior part of the vertebral body showing areas of demineralization and loss of margin contour. Findings of next vertebral involvement are common. Sclerotic changes persist but the rest of the vertebra remains without involvement [36]. Although the disk is commonly obliterated, collected data show that multiple sites and sparing of the disk are possible [37].

Arthritis may occur as part of direct infectious process to the joint or due to an inflammatory response. The infectious process is monoarticular and may affect any joint but most commonly the hip. The symptoms progress from weeks to months and presents with chronic swelling, pain, and loss of function without erythema. Constitutional symptoms occur in less than 30% of the cases [38]. The joint presents with effusion and loss of function with associated granulomatous changes, such changes lead to distortion and deformity of the joint. Treatment may include total hip replacement if debridement and antituberculous treatment is given [39]. Prosthetic joints can also be affected but it is very rarely. While arthroplasty may have an adequate outcome, infections related to hardware may co-exist with other bacterial infections. The same is painful, and hardware needs to be removed. On the other hand, symmetrical polyarthritis may involve large and small joints without local evidence of active TB, despite the presence of military, pulmonary, or extrapulmonary manifestations of the disease. Poncet's disease, other name given to the condition, seems to be immune-mediated and related to HIV co-infection. The inflammation resolves after starting antitubercular treatment without evidence of joint destruction [40]. Phemister triad may be observed in this case. The same consists of juxta-articular osteopenia or osteoporosis, peripheral osseous erosions, and gradual narrowing of the joint space. Although there is also evidence of local swelling and bode destruction, there is a preservation of the cartilage space.

Osteomyelitis may occur in any bone of the body, and it is more commonly insidious but the case has described acute and subacute onsets, which are very rare.

Clinical scenarios may include suspected malignancies or metastasis, but those findings are due to lytic tubercular lesions. It presents in unusual areas such as symphysis pubis, elbow, and sacroiliac joint [41]. Small bones may be affected without evidence of active pulmonary disease [38]. Ribs and sternum may also be affected. The firs may be confused as a breast or chest wall mass. The second may occur after coronary bypass surgery due to previous mediastinal involvement or as primary focus [42]. Radiological evident is usually present at the time of clinical presentation. There is osteolytic changes with minimal or none inflammatory changes, periarticular osteopenia, soft tissue swelling, and minimal or periosteal elevation [43].

Musculoskeletal involvement may also be seen at the epidural space, as an extraspinal mass or psoas abscess. The presentation may cause cord compression, rib erosion, and sinus tracts to the groin, respectively.

The diagnosis of musculoskeletal tuberculosis is challenging considering its indolent progression and clinical presentation. Caliceal suspicion is warrant and detail travel history and exposition in needed. In addition, although, a chest X-ray neither includes nor excludes the presence of extrapulmonary manifestation, and it may give a clue of current situation or evidence of previous infection. Other studies such as computer tomography, myelography, and MRI help to describe in detail joint and spinal cord involvement. Biopsy with microscopy and culture of the suspected or infected area is need for drug testing and identification of isolates. Synovial biopsy is needed in case of TB arthritis is considered. The fluid may be aspirate and verified but findings and usually nonspecific. In case of findings or with draining sinus, culture of the latter may help to identify the pathogen, although polymicrobial isolates and fungal results may be present and misleading [44].

Treatment is very similar to pulmonary TB. However, the course of therapy relies in whether the drug regime includes rifampin or not. Data suggest that dose that include rifampin may be shorter and as equally as effective as longer treatments (6–9 vs. 9–12 months). Shorter courses such as 6 months may be suitable on those cases that involve radical surgical resections [45]. Also, randomized clinical trials show comparable results after 5 years of treatment on those patients who received isoniazid with rifampin for 6–9 months vs. those who received isoniazid with either paraminosalicylic acid or ethambutol. Sixteen surgeries are required in different settings such as chest wall abscess, spinal diseases with a kyphosis of more than 40°, and spinal disease with progressive neurological deficits while on treatment or just advance neurological deterioration. This would lead to different alternatives such as decompression, drainage, debridement, and hardware placement for spine stabilization [46].

6.7 Cutaneous manifestations of tuberculosis

Although uncommon, tuberculosis also has skin manifestations. The same have been documented since 1826 and occurs in 1–2% of the infected individuals. Cutaneous classification varies, and it depends not only on clinical appearance but also on the method of infection, predisposing factors, and pre-existing TB exposure. The bacterial load may be variable, the same may be easily or difficult to detect [47]. Mode of infection may be due to inoculation secondary to exogenous source, endogenous (continue infection), or hematogenous spread.

Exogenous inoculation can occur due to primary inoculation or due to tuberculosis verrucosa cutis (TBVC). Primary inoculation is rare and occurs after direct skin invasion of a previous nonsensitized patient. Children of endemic areas are more affected. However, surgical procedure with infected equipment, piercing, and tattoos has been identified as causals. The infection is clinically apparent by the fourth week. A painless brown papule or nodule shallow about 1 cm affecting the

face and extremities. The lesion progresses slowly, and regional painless lymphadenopathy develops. The same may cause sinus draining tracks following skin perfora-
tion. Diagnosis relies on the tissue sample, acid fast, and culture. If left untreated,
the patient became sensitize to tuberculin test. Hematogenous spread is possible
resulting military pattern [48].

On the other hand, TBVC occurs after direct inoculation in a patient who is already
sensitized with TB. Children of endemic areas are at high risk and those who are occu-
pationally related. In children, the buttocks and ankles are more commonly affected,
while in adults, it occurs more frequently at the fingers and the dorsum of the hands.
It also presents with red-brown painless but warty plaques that grows peripherally.
Ulceration and regional lymphadenopathy is not common, it may co-exist with bacterial infection. Diagnose may be challenge. Culture form the lesion are usually negative,
tuberculin test is positive, and interferon gamma assay may play a role in the diagnosis.
Biopsy superficial dermal pseudoepitheliomatous hyperplasia with hyperkeratosis and
microabscess in the dermis or pseudoepitheliomatous rete pegs. The upper and middle
dermis shows inflammatory infiltrates of giant and epithelioid cells. Patient usually
responds to anti-TB treatment. If left untreated, lesions may persist [49].

Cutaneous involvement may also be causes by contiguous spread presenting as
Scrofuloderma, tuberculosis cutis orificialis, and lupus vulgaris. Scrofuloderma
are painless red-brown nodules subcutaneously located most commonly at the
axillar, neck, and groin areas. The infection occurs because of direct extension of
the infection from deeps structures invading the skin. Cervical nodes are the most
common site of infection. They tend to enlarge forming ulcers and sinus tracts and
may follow a line lymphoid distribution. Although the infection has been related to
Mycobacterium tuberculosis, it has been described in other in mycobacterial infections other than tuberculosis such as bovis and following BCG vaccination [49].
The lesion may be healed spontaneously, but it may take a long time to leave a scar.
Lupus vulgaris may be developed in association to the later. Children, adolescents,
and older adults are more commonly affected. Diagnosis is made by smear, culture,
and biopsy. Tuberculin test is usually positive, and concomitant pulmonary disease
is common [50].

Tuberculosis cutis orificialis (TBCO) is a rare manifestation of characterized by
painful ulcers with pseudomembranous fibrous base from a prior red-yellow nodule
with associated inflammation. The lesion may be sited at the oral, nasal, or anogenital
area. It affects middle age and older adults with advance immunodeficient disease (cell-
mediated). Most of these patients already have a progressive, pulmonary, gastrointestinal, or genitourinary advance TB disease. Tuberculin test is usually positive. Clinical
course is usually poor leading to disseminated military TB. Diagnosis relies on biopsy
smear and bacilli identification with the identification of them at the ulcer. The same is
also associated with tubercular granulomas at the edge of the ulcer and deep dermis.

Lupus vulgaris results as a manifestation of TB reactivation. Is a chronic manifestation that can occur by direct extension, lymphatics, or hematogenous spread?
It occurs more frequently on females than males, and it is the most common for old
TB skin manifestation in Europe. Despite this, it has a different distribution which
varies with geographical location. For example, in western countries, the distribution
is more common located at the head and neck areas, while in subtropical or tropical
areas is more common at the lower extremities [49]. The skin lesion is red-brown
papule that progresses into a nonpainful plaque. The same grows up to 10 cm developing areas of atrophy with associated central clearing. There are also variations of
the lesion, where it can develop hypertrophy and ulcerations. It may also infect with
other infections. As can be appreciated in other forms of granulomatous disease,
lesion can have a yellow-brown contour with "apple jelly" appearance [49]. Diagnosis
may be difficult, since it cannot be detected by culture or histopathology. PCR plays

a role in the identification of the mycobacteria. Although some cases have described, *Mycobacterium bovis* has potential pathogen. Pathology will show tuberculoid granulomas with central caseated lesions at the dermal area. The epidermal area may reveal atrophy acanthosis, hyperkeratosis. The disease, also known as Lupus TB, requires the use of anti Tb treatment. If not, the size of the lesion progresses developing ulceration of the skin with loss of architecture. Also, progression to skin-related cancer, such as squamous cell carcinoma, has been documented [50].

Skin lesion may also result from hematogenous spread from primary site of infection leading to metastatic tuberculous abscess, acute military TB, or lupus vulgaris. The first, metastatic tuberculous abscess occurs after developing cell-mediated immunodeficiency occurring in adults and malnourished children. The abscess may be single or multiple forms subcutaneous nontender nodules that progress to ulcer and sinus tract formation without lymphadenopathy [49, 51]. Any part of the skin may be affected more commonly the extremities. The metastatic infection usually confers a poor prognosis in the predispose individuals. Diagnosis is done after the findings of bacillus formation in culture, smears, or biopsies. Histopathological, there is evidence of ample skin necrosis, may show granulomas at the dermis. Unfortunately, tuberculin test results are variable [51].

Acute miliary TB is a rare manifestation that occurs more frequently in patients with deficient cell-mediated immunity such as infants and acquired immunodeficiency syndrome. Lesions are pinpoint red-bluish or purpuric papules with associated vesicles that furtherly become crusted. The lesion may resolve in the following weeks leaving hypopigmented scar like tissue. Skin biopsy plays a role in the diagnosis where mycobacteria are frequently identified. TST is usually negative [51].

Patient who have a higher immunity may develop hypersensitivity reaction manifestation as tuberculid. The lesions may be papulonecrotic, lichen scrofulosorum, and erythema induratum of Bazin (EIB). The identification of a tuberculid is supported after the following: presence of detectable infection such a TST and interferon gamma release assay, identification of granulomatous lesion in the skin, failure to identify *Mycobacterium tuberculosis* in cultures and stains, and noted, the resolution of the skin lesions after anti-Tb treatment.

Papulonecrotic tuberculid is the most common. It occurs more frequently in children and young adults. It is a dark violaceous papule that progress to pustular and necrosis. It is more commonly located in the face, neck, extremities extensor areas, and buttocks. It may be recurrent if left without treatment [51]. Constitutional symptoms occur prior the lesions and lymphadenitis can be appreciated [51]. The lesions may resolve alone leaving residual scars. Diagnosis is based on history of TB and evidence of wedge necrosis at the dermal and epidermal areas with granulomatous inflammation, mycobacterial DNA identification, and probable focus. TST is usually positive, and lesion resolves with anti-TB treatment.

Lichen scrofulosorum is rare and presents more frequently in children and young adult with previous infection at the lung, bone, lymph nodes, or intracranial. The lesion is small 1–5 mm red-brown -yellow commonly located at the truncal area [49, 51]. The lesions may resolve spontaneously without treatment. It does not leave a scar, and anti-TB treatment brings complete resolution. As other tuberculid, the diagnosis is based on clinical presentation, histopathologic findings (tuberculid granulomas at the upper dermis and tuber, glands, and hair follicles). TST is usually positive with negative mycobacterial culture.

Panniculitis of the lower extremity (EIB) may be seen in patients with TB. The manifestation usually occurs in middle age young females. The lesion is tender, red, subcutaneously located at the posterior aspects of the leg. The nodules may progress forming draining ulcers. Its course is chronic and resolves alone leaving scars. Anti-TB treatment is recommended. If panniculitis is associated to TB, TST is often positive. Diagnosis is based on clinical history and histopathological findings. Mycobacterial DNA may be identified by PCR but not always. Biopsy needs to include subcutaneous fat in a wedge fashion. The sample should reveal lobular with or without septal panniculitis, poorly form granulomas, necrosis of the fat with mixed inflammatory cells. Vasculitis may also. Other treatment alternatives include colchicine, NSAID's, potassium iodide, dapsone, tetracyclines, and antimalarial. Other kind of tuberculid, similar to EIB, is the nodular pattern occurs at the same areas but the granulomatous findings occur at the dermal-subcutaneous fat junction without ulceration or evidence of panniculitis.

7. Conclusions

Tuberculosis can invade almost any organ through the lymphatic system and blood dissemination. The manifestations of extra pulmonary tuberculosis can be variable depending on the organ and the system involved. The diagnosis is made through a high suspicion in the predisposed populations, and many times, extensive diagnostic tests that usually involve cultures and/or biopsies of the infected tissue. This is one of the infectious affections with a greater range of presentations, capable of pretending to be other noninfectious diagnoses.

Conflict of interest

No conflict of interest.

Author details

Onix J. Cantres-Fonseca*, William Rodriguez-Cintrón, Francisco Del Olmo-Arroyo and Stella Baez-Corujo
Veterans Affairs Caribbean Health System, San Juan, Puerto Rico

*Address all correspondence to: onixcantres@gmail.com

IntechOpen

References

[1] Elder NC. Extrapulmonary tuberculosis. A review. Archives of Family Medicine. 1992;**1**(1):91-98

[2] Binesh F, Zahir ST, Bovanlu TR. Isolated cerebellar tuberculoma mimicking posterior cranial fossa tumour. BML Case Reports. 2013

[3] Global Tuberculosis Report 2017. Wold Health Organization

[4] Mazza-Stadler J, Nicod L. Extra pulmonary tuberculosis. Revue des Maladies Respiratoires. 2012;**29**(4):566-578

[5] Kulchavenya E. Extrapulmonary tuberculosis: Are statistical reports accurate? Therapeutic Advances in Infectious Disease. 2014;**2**(2):61-70

[6] García-Rodríguez JF, Álvarez-Díaz H, Lorenzo-García M, Mariño-Callejo A, Fernández-Rial A, Sesma-Sánchez P. Extrapulmonary tuberculosis: Epidemiology and risk factors. Enfermedades Infecciosas y Microbiología Clínica. 2011;**29**(7):502-509

[7] Ates Gulera S, Mehmet B, Incic Omer F, Kokoglua Hasan F, Sevinc Ozdend U, Yukselc M. Evaluation of pulmonary and extrapulmonary tuberculosis in immunocompetent adults: A retrospective case series analysis. Medical Principles and Practice. 2014;**24**:75-79

[8] Peto H, Pratt RH, Harrington TA, Loblue P, Amstrong L. Epidemiology of extrapulmonary tuberculosis in the United States, 1993-2006. Clinical Infectious Diseases. 2009;**49**(9):1350-1357

[9] Lin JN, Lai CH, Chen YH, Lee SS, Tsai SS, Huang CK, et al. Risk factors for extra-pulmonary tuberculosis compared to pulmonary tuberculosis. The International Journal of Tuberculosis and Lung Disease. 2009;**5**:1350-1357

[10] Rock B, Olin M, Baker C, Molitor T, Peterson P. Central nervous system tuberculosis: Pathogenesis and clinical aspects. Clinical Microbiology Reviews. 2008;**21**(2):243-261

[11] Gomes da Rocha Dias A, Amann B, Costeira J, Gomes C, Bárbara C. Extrapulmonary tuberculosis in HIV infected patients admitted to the hospital. The European Respiratory Journal. 2016;**48**:PA2761

[12] Kneche NA. Tuberculosis: Pathophysiology, clinical features, and diagnosis. Critical Care Nurse. 2009;**29**(2):34-43

[13] Burke HE. A new approach to the pathogenesis of extrapulmonary tuberculosis. The British Journal of Tuberculosis and Diseases of the Chest. 1954;**48**(1):3-11

[14] Cherian A, Thomas SV. Central nervous system tuberculosis. African Health Sciences. 2011;**11**(1):116-127

[15] Yaramiş A, Gurkan F, Elevli M, Söker M, Haspolat K, Kirbaş G, et al. Central nervous system tuberculosis in children: A review of 214 cases. Pediatrics. 1998;**102**(5):1-5

[16] Sütlaş PN, Unal A, Forta H, Senol S, Kirbas D. Tuberculous meningitis in adults: Review of 61 cases. Infection. 2003;**31**(6):387-391

[17] Monteiro R, Carneiro JC, Duarte R. Cerebral tuberculomas – A clinical challenge. Respiratory Medicine Case Reports Elsevier. 2013;**9**:34-37

[18] Vorster MJ, Allwood B, Koegelenberg C. Tuberculous pleural effusions: Advances and controversies. Cochrane Database of Systematic Reviews. 2016

[19] FORMATEX 2013. The Challenge of Diagnosing Pleural Tuberculosis

Infection. Microbial pathogens and strategies for combating them: Science, technology and education (A. Méndez-Vilas, Ed.): http://www.formatex.info/microbiology4/vol3/1950-1956.pdf

[20] Kirsch CM, Kroe DM, Azzi RL, Jensen WA, Kagawa FT, Wehner JH. The optimal number of pleural biopsy specimens for a diagnosis of tuberculous pleurisy. Chest. 1997;**112**(3):702-706

[21] Tripathi PB, Amarapurkar AD. Morphological spectrum of gastrointestinal tuberculosis. Tropical Gastroenterology. 2009;**30**(1):35-39

[22] Lin PY, Wang JY, Hsueh PR, Lee LN, Hsiao CH, Yu CJ, et al. Lower gastrointestinal tract tuberculosis: An important but neglected disease. International Journal of Colorectal Disease. 2009;**24**(10):1175-1180

[23] Park SH, Yang SK, Yang DH, Kim KJ, Yoon SM, Choe JW, et al. Prospective randomized trial of six-month versus nine-month therapy for intestinal tuberculosis. Antimicrobial Agents and Chemotherapy. 2009;**53**(10):4167-4171

[24] Williford ME, Thompson WM, Hamilton JD. Esophageal tuberculosis: Findings on barium swallow and computed tomography. Gastrointestinal Radiology. 1983;**8**(2):119-122

[25] Ozbülbül NI, Ozdemir M, Turhan N. CT findings in fatal primary intestinal tuberculosis in a liver transplant recipient. Diagnostic and Interventional Radiology. 2008;**14**(4):221-224

[26] Brown LP, Nelson AM, Brown AE, et al. Gastrointestinal manifestations of acquired immunodeficiency syndrome. Radiological Society of North America; 1995. Available at: http://www.rsna.org/REG/publications/rg/afip/privateM/1995/0015/00

[27] Radin DR. Intraabdominal *Mycobacterium tuberculosis* vs

Mycobacterium avium-intracellulare infections in patients with AIDS: Distinction based on CT findings. AJR. American Journal of Roentgenology. 1991;**156**(3):487-491

[28] Epstein BM, Mann JH. CT of abdominal tuberculosis. AJR. American Journal of Roentgenology. 1982;**139**(5):861-866

[29] Yang ZG, Min PQ, Sone S. Tuberculosis versus lymphomas in the abdominal lymph nodes: Evaluation with contrast-enhanced CT. AJR. American Journal of Roentgenology. 1999;**172**(3):619-623

[30] Zajaczkowski T. Genitourinary tuberculosis: Historical and basic science review: Past and present. Central European Journal of Urology. 2012;**65**(4):182-187

[31] Eastwood J. Tuberculosis and the kidney. JASN. 2001;**12**(6):1307-1314

[32] Hershkovitz I, Donoghue HD, Minnikin DE, et al. Detection and molecular characterization of 9,000-year-old *Mycobacterium tuberculosis* from a Neolithic settlement in the eastern Mediterranean. PLoS One. 2008;**3**:e3426

[33] Watts HG, Lifeso RM. Tuberculosis of bones and joints. The Journal of Bone and Joint Surgery. American Volume. 1996;**78**:288

[34] Ellner JJ. Review: The immune response in human tuberculosis--implications for tuberculosis control. The Journal of Infectious Diseases. 1997;**176**:1351

[35] Lenaerts A, Barry CE 3rd, Dartois V. Heterogeneity in tuberculosis pathology, microenvironments and therapeutic responses. Immunological Reviews. 2015;**264**:288

[36] Polley P, Dunn R. Noncontiguous spinal tuberculosis: Incidence and

management. European Spine Journal. 2009;**18**:1096

[37] Yao DC, Sartoris DJ. Musculoskeletal tuberculosis. Radiologic Clinics of North America. 1995;**33**:679

[38] Pertuiset E, Beaudreuil J, Lioté F, et al. Spinal tuberculosis in adults. A study of 103 cases in a developed country, 1980-1994. Medicine (Baltimore). 1999;**78**:309

[39] Hodgson SP, Ormerod LP. Ten-year experience of bone and joint tuberculosis in Blackburn 1978-1987. Journal of the Royal College of Surgeons of Edinburgh. 1990;**35**:259

[40] Kim SJ, Postigo R, Koo S, Kim JH. Total hip replacement for patients with active tuberculosis of the hip: A systematic review and pooled analysis. The Bone & Joint Journal. 2013;**95-B**:578

[41] Arora S, Prakash TV, Carey RA, Hansdak SG. Poncet's disease: Unusual presentation of a common disease. Lancet. 2016;**387**:617

[42] Karanas YL, Yim KK. *Mycobacterium tuberculosis* infection of the hand: A case report and review of the literature. Annals of Plastic Surgery. 1998;**40**:65

[43] Platt MA, Ziegler K. Primary sternal osteomyelitis with bacteremia and distal seeding. The Journal of Emergency Medicine. 2012;**43**:e93

[44] Shikhare SN, Singh DR, Shimpi TR, Peh WC. Tuberculous osteomyelitis and spondylodiscitis. Seminars in Musculoskeletal Radiology. 2011;**15**(5):446-458

[45] Colmenero JD, Ruiz-Mesa JD, Sanjuan-Jimenez R, et al. Establishing the diagnosis of tuberculous vertebral osteomyelitis. European Spine Journal. 2013;**22**(Suppl 4):579

[46] Upadhyay SS, Sell P, Saji MJ, et al. Surgical management of spinal tuberculosis in adults. Hong Kong operation compared with debridement surgery for short and long term outcome of deformity. Clinical Orthopaedics and Related Research. 1994;**302**:173

[47] Bravo FG, Gotuzzo E. Cutaneous tuberculosis. Clinics in Dermatology. 2007;**25**:173

[48] MacGregor RR. Cutaneous tuberculosis. Clinics in Dermatology. 1995;**13**:245

[49] Tappeiner G. Tuberculosis and infections with atypical mycobacteria. In: Wolff K, Goldsmith LA, Katz SI, et al., editors. Fitzparick's Dermatology in General Medicine. 7th ed. New York: McGraw Hill Medical; 2008. p. 1768

[50] Kanitakis J, Audeffray D, Claudy A. Squamous cell carcinoma of the skin complicating lupus vulgaris. Journal of the European Academy of Dermatology and Venereology. 2006;**20**:114

[51] Barbagallo J, Tager P, Ingleton R, et al. Cutaneous tuberculosis: Diagnosis and treatment. American Journal of Clinical Dermatology. 2002;**3**:319